THIRD EDITION

CATARACTS
A Patient's Guide to Treatment

THIRD EDITION

CATARACTS
A Patient's Guide to Treatment

David F. Chang, MD
Altos Eye Physicians
Los Altos, California

Bryan S. Lee, MD, JD
Altos Eye Physicians
Los Altos, California

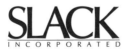

www.Healio.com/books

ISBN: 978-1-63091-215-4

Copyright © 2016 by SLACK Incorporated

A previous edition of *Cataracts: A Patient's Guide to Treatment* was published by Addicus Books.

Dr. David F. Chang and Dr. Bryan S. Lee have no financial or proprietary interest in the materials presented herein.

The procedures and practices described in this publication should be implemented in a manner consistent with the professional standards set for the circumstances that apply in each specific situation. Every effort has been made to confirm the accuracy of the information presented and to correctly relate generally accepted practices. The authors, editors, and publisher cannot accept responsibility for errors or exclusions or for the outcome of the material presented herein. There is no expressed or implied warranty of this book or information imparted by it. Care has been taken to ensure that drug selection and dosages are in accordance with currently accepted/recommended practice. Off-label uses of drugs may be discussed. Due to continuing research, changes in government policy and regulations, and various effects of drug reactions and interactions, it is recommended that the reader carefully review all materials and literature provided for each drug, especially those that are new or not frequently used. Some drugs or devices in this publication have clearance for use in a restricted research setting by the Food and Drug and Administration or FDA. Each professional should determine the FDA status of any drug or device prior to use in their practice.

Any review or mention of specific companies or products is not intended as an endorsement by the author or publisher.

SLACK Incorporated uses a review process to evaluate submitted material. Prior to publication, educators or clinicians provide important feedback on the content that we publish. We welcome feedback on this work.

Published by: SLACK Incorporated
                       6900 Grove Road
                       Thorofare, NJ 08086 USA
                       Telephone: 856-848-1000
                       Fax: 856-848-6091
                       www.Healio.com/books

Contact SLACK Incorporated for more information about other books in this field or about the availability of our books from distributors outside the United States.

Library of Congress Cataloging-in-Publication Data

Names: Chang, David F., 1954- author. | Lee, Bryan S., author.
Title: Cataracts : a patient's guide to treatment / David F. Chang, MD, Bryan
    S. Lee, MD, JD.
Description: Third edition. | Thorofare, NJ : Slack Incorporated, [2016] |
    Includes index.
Identifiers: LCCN 2016010980 (print) | ISBN 9781630912154 (paperback)
Subjects: LCSH: Cataract--Surgery. | Patient education. | BISAC: MEDICAL /
    Ophthalmology.
Classification: LCC RE451 .C43 2016 (print) | DDC 617.7/42059--dc23
LC record available at http://lccn.loc.gov/2016010980

Printed in the United States of America.

Last digit is print number: 10 9 8 7 6 5 4 3 2

Dedication

To our dedicated staff at
Peninsula Eye Surgery Center and at
Altos Eye Physicians, some of whom have worked in
our office for more than 30 years. We are grateful for
your daily, tireless efforts in helping to educate and
care for our patients.

Contents

Introduction

If you have picked up this book, perhaps you're worried that you have a cataract. Maybe your vision has become blurry, or you feel as if you're looking through mist or a lace curtain. You may find yourself backing away from some of your favorite activities, such as reading, work, or hobbies that require good vision. Perhaps you have difficulty seeing when you're driving at night. If you are experiencing such vision problems, you may have a cataract—the most common vision problem in the United States.

The good news is that cataract surgery can restore your vision. Helping people regain vision they have lost is one of the most gratifying experiences that a physician can have. Having steered many thousands of patients through this procedure, we have an appreciation for a patient's most common concerns and fears.

Because we know that the thought of surgery on your eyes may make you feel anxious, we have written this book to help you understand cataracts and allay your concerns. We will explain how cataracts form, how they're diagnosed, and how they're treated. We will also discuss follow-up care and special conditions that may affect cataract surgery. We believe that with this knowledge, you'll be better equipped to talk with your doctor about the best way to improve your vision. It is important that you're able to make an informed decision about cataract treatment that could make your world bright and clear once again.

Dr. David F. Chang

Dr. Bryan S. Lee

Chapter 1

How the Human Eye Works

"I just don't see as well as I used to."

You might have said these words in frustration as you tried to thread a needle or do a crossword puzzle. Maybe you've given up driving at night or started using a magnifying glass to read. Reading might not be as enjoyable as it once was, or it may be more difficult to see details on the television screen. It might seem as though you continually need new eyeglass or contact lens prescriptions.

Of course, you're concerned. Of all our senses, sight may be the one we most rely on. We depend on our eyes for the ability to move about freely—to walk, drive, dance, or bicycle. Our eyes keep us mobile and independent. When your eyes transmit images to the brain, they supply a perpetual stream of information from the world around you.

Chang DF, Lee BS.
Cataracts: A Patient's Guide to Treatment,
Third Edition (pp 1-9).
© 2016 SLACK Incorporated.

Figure 1-1. The image demonstrates the similarities between a camera and the eyeball.

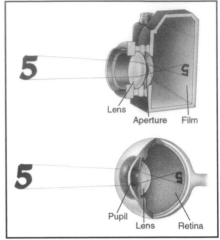

Anatomy of the Eye

You've probably heard it said that the eye works much like a camera. It focuses light to form images and then converts those images into nerve impulses for the brain to interpret. This is similar to the way a camera lens transmits images to film (Figure 1-1).

The eyes are spheres about an inch in diameter—self-lubricating, self-cleansing, well-protected, and so sensitive that they can distinguish between images only one ten-thousandth of an inch apart. An eyeball is made up of several complex parts (Figure 1-2).

The *sclera* forms the round wall of the eyeball, the part we commonly refer to as the white of the eye. The sclera is a tough, thick, opaque structure that protects the delicate structures inside the eyeball.

The *conjunctiva* is a thin mucous membrane that covers the sclera; this transparent membrane, along with the eyelids, protects your eyeball from environmental irritants.

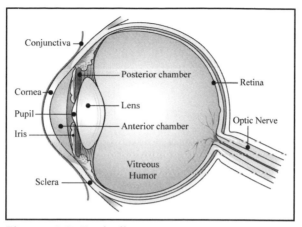

Figure 1-2. Eyeball anatomy.

The *cornea* is a transparent, dome-like window at the front of the eye. As light enters your eye, the cornea bends, or refracts, the light before it passes through the lens. Unlike most other structures in your body, the cornea contains no blood vessels; instead, it receives oxygen from the air and other nourishment from the aqueous humor, a clear liquid between the cornea and lens. (The aqueous humor also keeps your eyeball inflated at the proper pressure.) Because it is rich in nerve fibers, the cornea is very sensitive. This is why you feel even the tiniest foreign object, such as dust or an eyelash, when it lands on your eye's surface.

The *iris* is the part of the eye we refer to when we describe the color of someone's eyes. Typically a shade of brown or blue, the iris sits behind the cornea and acts like a curtain as it controls the amount of light entering the eye.

The *pupil* is the black hole in the center of your iris that allows light to enter the eye. In low light, the muscles of the iris cause the pupil to open wide, or dilate, to permit more light to enter; likewise, the pupil constricts in bright light.

The *lens*, which sits just behind the pupil, is a flexible structure made of clear protein that helps focus light onto your retina. Surrounded by a thin membrane called the *capsule* or *capsular bag*, the lens is shaped like an M&M candy. It changes shape—flattening or thickening to bring objects at various distances into focus—in a process called *accommodation*. The lens loses flexibility over time, and by our early 40s, most of us find that it's harder for our eyes to shift focus.

The *retina* lines the back half of your eyeball. About the size of a postage stamp and as thin as an onion skin, the retina is the "film" of the camera. It registers light images and sends them to your brain through a bundle of nerve fibers called the *optic nerve*. Your brain then "develops the film," interpreting the shapes, colors, and details of the images it receives.

The cavity between the lens and the retina is filled with a transparent, gel-like substance called the *vitreous humor*, through which light rays pass. As this gel becomes more watery with age, tiny residual solid portions can move. This creates harmless drifting shadows that may appear as veils or floaters.

How the Eyes Stay Lubricated

In a marvelous process provided by nature, the surface of your eyes is constantly lubricated and rinsed by a steady production of tears. Tears flow from glands at the outer, upper corners of each eye and drain through tiny tear ducts located in the upper and lower inner corners of our eyelids. When we blink, we pump tears from the eye surface into the tear duct drainage system. This is why if we are about to cry, we start to blink more as our eyes are welling up with tears. Rapid blinking pumps the tears into the tear ducts.

The tear ducts pass through channels within the bones of the nose and eventually empty the tears into the back of your throat. This also explains the otherwise puzzling phenomenon of being able to taste eye drops.

Common Vision Problems

REFRACTIVE ERRORS

There are 2 basic causes of blurred vision: refractive error and eye disease. Refractive errors are common, naturally occurring optical imperfections that are easily treated with glasses or contact lenses. Four common examples are described below. People with good distance eyesight naturally have optically normal eyes (Figure 1-3). Their eyes naturally focus light rays sharply onto the retina.

> *Refractive errors are common, naturally occurring optical imperfections that are easily treated with glasses or contact lenses.*

Nearsightedness (myopia) occurs when the eye bends light too soon, focusing the rays in front of rather than on the retina (Figure 1-4). If you're myopic, you see nearby objects better than you see objects that are far away. Images in the distance appear blurry.

Farsightedness (hyperopia) occurs when the eye bends light too late, focusing the rays "behind" the retina (Figure 1-5). If you're farsighted, both far and near images appear blurry, but closer objects are much blurrier than farther objects.

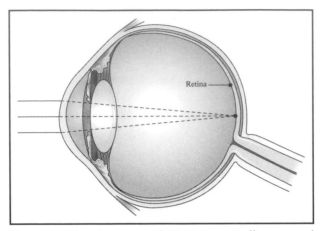

Figure 1-3. When one has an optically normal eye, light rays enter through the cornea and lens and strike the retina, producing a focused image.

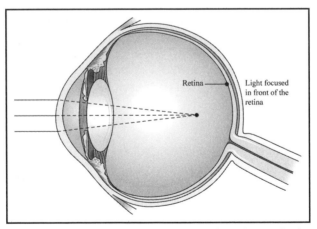

Figure 1-4. In myopia, or nearsightedness, light rays focus in front of the retina, causing distant objects to appear blurry.

Presbyopia is a result of normal age-related changes in the lens, which becomes less flexible over time. As the lens stiffens, the eye muscles responsible for accommodation

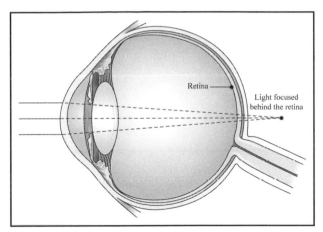

Figure 1 5. In hyperopia, or farsightedness, light rays focus behind the retina. Objects in the distance are blurry, but not as blurry as near objects.

can no longer change the lens shape enough to focus on close objects. If you're in your 40s or older, you've probably experienced this unavoidable condition. You may have started wearing reading glasses or bifocals to compensate for the loss of your natural focusing ability.

Astigmatism occurs when the cornea's curvature is oblong like the back of a spoon instead of rounded like a basketball (Figure 1-6). This common refractive error blurs both far and near vision when glasses or contact lenses are not worn.

COMMON EYE DISORDERS

The second category of conditions that impair vision consists of abnormalities not correctable with glasses because they involve the vision-producing structures of the eye. Cataracts are one such condition; others are briefly introduced next and discussed in more detail in Chapter 9.

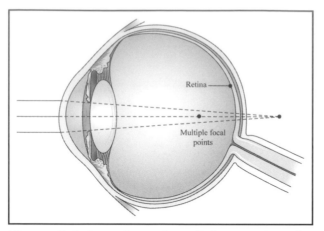

Figure 1-6. In astigmatism, light entering the eyeball focuses on multiple areas rather than on the retina. Objects both far and near appear blurry.

Macular degeneration is one of a dozen or so conditions that can affect the retina. A painless disorder common among older people, macular degeneration is caused by age-related deterioration of the central part of the retina, the macula. Macular degeneration may cause a gradual deterioration of central vision. Although it is a potentially serious problem, the majority of patients will not suffer severe vision loss. There is a wide spectrum in the severity of the problem, however.

Glaucoma, which also occurs more often as we age, is a condition in which the pressure of the fluid in the eye becomes too high, causing damage to the optic nerve. If diagnosed early enough, glaucoma can be treated with eye drops or surgery to lower the fluid pressure, such as by helping it to drain more quickly from the eye. Left untreated, glaucoma can irrevocably damage the optic nerve and lead to blindness.

Diabetic retinopathy refers to circulation problems in the retina that result from years of elevated blood sugar. Fluid may leak from diseased blood vessels into the retina, or abnormal vessels in the retina may bleed into the vitreous cavity. Although laser treatments, medications, or surgery can help, it is better to prevent these problems through consistent control of the blood sugar level.

Other health conditions can cause blurry vision, so see your doctor if you experience a reduction in the clarity of your vision. The right diagnosis and proper treatment can protect your eyes and preserve—or improve—your vision.

Chapter 2

Understanding Cataracts

I f you've reached your 60s, you have probably begun to feel some of the effects of aging on your vision. Most of us are not seeing as well as we once did, and cataracts may be a factor. In fact, for those over the age of 40, cataracts are one of the most common reasons for poor eyesight. Cataracts are the most common cause of reversible vision loss in the United States. In developing countries, where cataract surgery is often unavailable, cataracts are the leading cause of blindness.

Most cataracts occur as a result of aging. These cataracts often begin in one's 40s or 50s, but they may not affect vision until after age 60. According to the

Cataracts are the most common cause of reversible vision loss in the United States. In developing countries, where cataract surgery is often unavailable, cataracts are the leading cause of blindness.

Chang DF, Lee BS.
Cataracts: A Patient's Guide to Treatment,
Third Edition (pp 11-20).
© 2016 SLACK Incorporated.

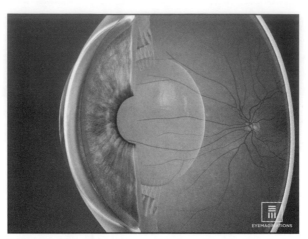

Figure 2-1. The natural lens sits behind the iris and should be clear.

American Academy of Ophthalmology (AAO), those between the ages of 52 and 64 have a 50/50 chance of developing a cataract. By age 75, nearly everyone has at least some cataract formation.

What Is a Cataract?

The word *cataract* comes from the Greek word for waterfall. It was once believed that a milky substance "falling" into the eye caused cataracts. Today, we know that a cataract is a gradual clouding of the eye's lens (Figures 2-1 and 2-2). How does this come about? The lens is made mostly of protein and water. Over time, the protein clumps together, creating a cloudiness in areas of the lens. As a result, light does not pass through the lens as well, and vision is affected.

There is often confusion about the relationship between the natural lens and a cataract. A cataract is not a growth on the lens; a cataract is the clouded lens itself.

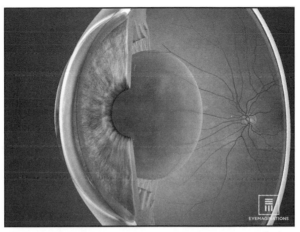

Figure 2-2. A cataract is a clouding of the natural lens that usually occurs with age.

Types of Cataracts

There are several basic types of cataracts. It is important to note that the type or location is not as important as the severity of a cataract. The severity, whether it is mild, moderate, or advanced, determines the need for corrective surgery. The type of cataract has no real bearing on the need for surgery.

- **Age-related cataracts** form as the eyeball ages.
- **Traumatic cataracts** develop after an eye injury (may be years later).
- **Congenital cataracts** appear in babies or develop in children, often in both eyes.

Cataracts can also be classified according to their location within the lens. Nuclear cataracts, the most common, form in the center of the lens. Cortical cataracts are spoke-like, beginning near the outer part of the lens and extending inward toward the center. Subcapsular cataracts begin at the very front or back of the lens; these cataracts in particular sometimes develop very quickly.

Symptoms of Cataracts

How do you know if you have a cataract? They usually can't be seen with the naked eye. They're painless; their progress is typically gradual; and they don't cause symptoms such as redness, discomfort, or tearing. The loss of visual acuity, or sharpness, in one or both eyes is progressive, but slow. Consequently, many people don't even realize they have a cataract at first. Individual symptoms vary greatly, depending on the severity, location, and type of cataract. Some people have trouble seeing in dim light or may experience difficulty reading street signs or small print (Figure CA-1). Occasionally, others may experience double vision in one eye. Some may notice a troublesome glare in bright sunlight or when facing oncoming headlights in traffic.

What are some indications that you may have a cataract? If you answer "yes" to several of the following questions, you may have cataracts:

- Is your vision blurry, cloudy, or foggy?
- Do you have trouble seeing distant details, such as highway signs or a golf ball?
- Do you need more light for close work?
- Do your eyes tire more easily when reading?
- Do you have trouble seeing in restaurants and other dimly lit rooms?
- Is your night vision poor?
- Does glare bother you, making it harder for you to drive at night or to see well in bright sunlight?
- Do you see ghost images, such as 2 or 3 moons at night?

- Do colors appear faded, washed out, or yellowish?
- Does your eyeglass prescription change frequently?

It is a common misconception that cataracts are visible to the naked eye. In fact, people often mistake whitish growths on the surface of the eye for cataracts, when that is not the case. Usually, these are callous-like growths that result from the cumulative effect of irritation caused by dryness and sunlight over many years. Similarly, as we age, we may develop a hazy white ring around the edges of the cornea. Many people think these rings are cataracts, but they are actually an accumulation of cholesterol deposited by nearby blood vessels. They do not affect vision and do not represent an abnormal cholesterol level. They simply are a sign of aging. Like gray hair, they have no real health significance.

How Cataracts Progress

In the early stages, cataracts may not cause vision problems. The cloudiness may affect only a small portion of the lens. However, over time the cloudiness increases, making vision worse (Figures 2-3 and 2-4). The speed with which cataracts progress varies greatly with each person. Typically, the initial mild symptoms will progress rather gradually, perhaps over the course of several years. However, the cataract may then start to change much more rapidly. It is impossible to predict when you will need surgery. Once vision begins to deteriorate more quickly, the need for surgery becomes quite obvious. Because cataracts are a result of normal aging, they eventually develop in both eyes, although one eye may develop a cataract earlier or more quickly than the other. This doesn't mean that the eye with the worse cataract is abnormal or in poorer health than the other eye. A cataract in one eye does not affect the health or function of the other eye.

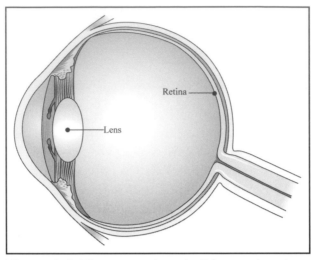

Figure 2-3. The normal eyeball has a clear lens through which light can pass.

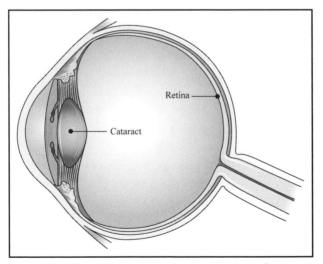

Figure 2-4. In this eye, a cataract has formed. Note how the lens has become cloudy.

Other than blurring your vision, cataracts do not damage or harm your eyes. So the decision to have surgery is based primarily on your symptoms and the degree to which they interfere with your day-to-day life. If you are not having trouble with normal activities and you are satisfied with your eyesight, there is no pressing need to have a cataract removed.

As the cataract progresses, the lens becomes cloudier and eventually opaque. If it is not removed, the cataract can eventually obscure all useful vision in the affected eye. This does not happen all at once, but rather occurs in stages (except in the case of traumatic cataracts that form soon after a severe eye injury). The most advanced cataracts, called *mature cataracts*, cause the entire lens to turn white. At this point, the eye is functionally blind. If your cataract is already very advanced, don't wait for it to become this severe before having it removed.

Causes and Risk Factors

Scientists don't know the precise biological mechanisms that cause cataracts. However, they are exploring the theory that age-related cataracts develop when certain eye proteins, called *alpha-crystallins*, fail as the eyes get older. Alpha-crystallins do the important work of protecting lens proteins; without them, the normally clear lens proteins would clump and lose their transparency. But like other body cells, alpha-crystallins can be damaged by so-called *free radicals* (also called *oxygenating agents*). Free radicals are charged, highly unstable molecule fragments that harm healthy cells. Over time, damage from free radicals may prevent alpha-crystallins from doing their protective job or use up the alpha-crystallins, and cataracts develop.

As mentioned, age is the greatest risk factor related to the onset of cataracts. Cataracts are the most common cause of blurred vision in people over the age of 50. There are several other risk factors that you also have no control over, including the following:

- **Family history.** In certain families, cataracts tend to occur at earlier ages. Knowing at what age your parents developed cataracts, however, doesn't necessarily tell you at what age you might expect them.

- **Medical disorders.** Being diabetic raises the risk of cataracts 3- to 4-fold. High blood sugar levels react with proteins in the eye, forming byproducts that accumulate in the lens. Treatments for some illnesses—such as radiation to the head and total-body radiation treatments for cancer—can also induce cataracts. Rarely do cataracts occur at birth or develop during early childhood. When they do, the cause is usually unknown. However, diseases, inherited disorders, and infections during pregnancy (such as rubella) can play a part.

- **Nearsightedness.** People with more severe myopia can develop cataracts at an earlier age and may need surgery by the time they are in their 40s or 50s.

- **Steroid use.** If you take systemic steroid medications over a long period of time for conditions such as asthma or emphysema, you're at increased risk for cataracts. Long-term use of high doses of inhaled steroids also increases the risk. This is not as true of lower doses.

- **Eye diseases.** Certain eye diseases such as chronic internal eye inflammation, called *uveitis* or *iritis*, are associated with cataracts. Some premature babies develop a retinal disease, called *retinopathy of prematurity*, during infancy; they are prone to developing cataracts in their 40s. Having a type of retinal surgery called a *vitrectomy* also accelerates cataract formation.

- **Eye injuries.** Severe trauma to the eye at any age can cause a cataract to develop, even many years later. Cataracts can be caused by sharp objects or metal particles that penetrate the eye or by blunt injuries, such as from the impact of a ball, a punch, or a firecracker explosion. Eye injuries are the leading cause of cataracts in children and adolescents.

Preventing Cataracts

Several large studies have looked at whether certain vitamin or mineral supplements can prevent or delay cataracts. Unfortunately, the results have been disappointing. One landmark study found that antioxidants have no effect on cataract prevention. Other studies show that certain nonprescription medications and eye drops touted as preventing cataracts are also ineffective.

You can, however, take some steps that may delay the progression of cataracts and protect your overall health as well:

- **Don't smoke.** Cataracts occur more frequently among smokers. The evidence is clear: Not smoking is the single most important measure you can take to prevent cataracts.

- **Eat fruits and vegetables.** There is some evidence that a diet with plenty of fruits and vegetables may delay the onset of cataracts.
- **Protect your eyes from excessive sun exposure.** A hat with a brim can reduce sunlight exposure to your eyes by 30% to 50%. Wear sunglasses outdoors and protective eye goggles in tanning booths.
- **Manage diabetes well.** Work with your doctor to keep your blood sugar under control.
- **Avoid eye injuries.** Wear protective goggles when performing tasks that could result in eye injury. According to the United States Eye Injury Registry, 40% of eye injuries occur in the home, 13% occur in industrial settings, and 13% occur during sporting activities. Blunt objects account for 31% of injuries, and sharp objects cause 18% of eye injuries. Other causes include vehicle crashes, BB and pellet guns, nails, hammering metal, fireworks, guns, falls, and explosions.

Figures 2-1 and 2-2 have been reprinted with permission from Eyemaginations.

Chapter 3

Getting a Diagnosis

In the early stages of cataracts, you may not notice any problem with your everyday activities such as reading, driving, or watching television. At first, you may be able to compensate for your vision loss by using different eyeglasses, a magnifying glass, a larger computer font, or stronger lighting. However, as cataracts progress, vision problems become worse. Accordingly, it is important to get a diagnosis to see if your problems are from cataract or another cause.

Role of Eye Care Specialists

OPHTHALMOLOGISTS

Several types of health professionals are involved in eye care. An ophthalmologist is a medical doctor who specializes in medical and surgical eye care. General ophthalmologists diagnose and treat eye problems, including

Chang DF, Lee BS.
Cataracts: A Patient's Guide to Treatment,
Third Edition (pp 21-29).
© 2016 SLACK Incorporated.

common conditions that require surgery, such as cataracts. They also perform vision examinations and prescribe eyeglasses and contact lenses. Specialist ophthalmologists undergo additional training and choose to specialize in the treatment and surgery of a particular part of the eye; for example, they may be retina specialists or cornea specialists.

Ophthalmologists have extensive training and education—at least 4 years of premedical college education, 4 years or more of medical school, a 1-year internship, and 3 years or more of specialized medical and surgical training in eye diseases.

OPTOMETRISTS

Optometrists are licensed to provide basic eye care services, including testing for refractive problems such as nearsightedness or astigmatism. They also diagnose eye conditions and diseases such as cataracts. These eye doctors also prescribe corrective lenses (glasses and contacts) and medications for some eye disorders. Optometrists do not perform surgery, but they may advise you about surgery. For example, your optometrist can diagnose your cataracts and help you decide whether or not you should consider having cataract surgery. He or she can also refer you to a qualified ophthalmologist for surgery.

Optometrists complete 2 to 4 years of undergraduate studies and 4 years of postgraduate optometry school in order to be licensed.

OPTICIANS

Although opticians are not involved with the diagnosis of cataracts or other diseases, it may be helpful to clarify the role they play in your eye care. Opticians design, finish, fit, and dispense eyeglasses and contact lenses based

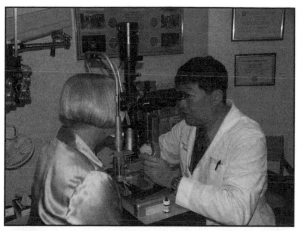

Figure 3-1. An eye doctor examines a patient using a slit lamp.

on an optometrist's or ophthalmologist's prescription. Opticians may also dispense colored and specialty lenses for special needs.

Your Appointment With an Eye Doctor

When you go to an eye specialist, he or she will perform a thorough examination, including a microscopic examination of the interior of your eyeballs (Figure 3-1). He or she will also perform a special examination designed to discover whether cataracts are present. During the examination, the doctor will ask questions about your eye history. This examination will be painless and can uncover other preventable or treatable problems that might damage your vision. During a complete eye examination, your doctor will do the following:

- Take your eye medical history
- Give you a vision test and check your eyeglass prescription

- Examine the exterior of your eyeballs
- Examine the interior of your eyeballs
- Measure the fluid pressure within your eyeballs

Your Eye and Medical History

Your doctor will want to know about any eye symptoms you are having. Try to be as accurate as possible when describing your symptoms. If your vision is impaired, explain which activities are difficult.

Your eye doctor will ask about your eye history and want to know when you had your last eye examination. You should mention any previous eye diseases, injuries, or surgeries you have had. List any prescription eye medications that you are taking. Also, tell your doctor if there is a history of glaucoma or retinal detachment in your family.

Your eye doctor needs to know about any major medical issues you may have. Common health problems such as diabetes, hypertension, heart disease, asthma, and emphysema can affect your eye health and impact treatment decisions. Your doctor will want to know about any prescription medications you are taking as well as allergies to medications. As will be explained in Chapter 9, it is important to mention if you have ever taken medications for an enlarged prostate.

Some medical problems can affect your comfort or your ability to cooperate during cataract surgery. Let your eye doctor know if you are hard of hearing; have claustrophobia, panic attacks, or sudden coughing attacks; or if you are allergic to latex. Also, let the doctor know if you have back pain, breathing problems, or any other condition that might make it difficult for you to lie flat.

Assessing Your Vision

One of the first things your eye doctor will want to do during your eye examination is assess your vision. If you're having difficulty seeing, you may have a health problem with your eye, or you may simply need glasses to correct your eye's inability to focus. Your doctor will want to assess your eyesight using a standard eye chart.

If you're having difficulty seeing, you may have a health problem with your eye, or you may simply need glasses to correct your eye's inability to focus.

What Is 20/20 Vision?

You've probably heard of 20/20 vision, but what exactly does it mean? This measure of visual acuity is based on how well you can read a vision chart from 20 feet away while you are wearing your glasses or contact lenses. The visual acuity chart, known as the *Snellen chart*, contains 12 to 13 rows of letters. The letters are largest in the top row and become progressively smaller with each descending row. Your visual acuity score is based on the smallest row of letters you are able to read.

Scores relate to how well someone with "perfect" vision reads the chart. For example, if your vision is 20/60 with your glasses on, it means you read the chart at 20 feet as well as someone with perfect vision could read it from 60 feet away.

Visual acuity can be tested with or without your eyeglasses. Your doctor will be more interested in your visual acuity score with your eyeglasses. Because healthy eyes should have excellent vision with the proper eyeglasses, testing your vision with your glasses on is the only way for your doctor to measure the effect of eye abnormalities such as cataracts and macular degeneration.

Although standard visual acuity tests are valuable, they do have limitations and do not address some types of vision problems cataracts may be causing. For example, the standard eye chart is not a good test for problems you may be having with contrast, color, glare, or peripheral vision.

Determining Refractive Error

If you are having difficulty seeing well at different distances without glasses, it is important to determine whether you simply need new eyeglasses or whether you have another problem, such as a cataract. As part of your eye examination, your doctor will need to determine your refractive error. This refers to natural imperfections in the optics of the eye that reduce how sharply images are focused onto your retina.

Because your vision problem may be solved with new glasses, your doctor will want to first determine the best eyeglass prescription for each of your eyes. This process, called the *refraction*, identifies, measures, and quantifies the refractive error in each eye. The results of the refraction will determine whether your lens prescription needs to be changed and, if so, by how much. Once your doctor has identified the best lens prescription for you, he or she will retest your ability to read the eye chart. If your vision is still abnormal, it indicates that you have a problem with the eye itself, and further testing is needed.

Examining the Eyeball

EXTERIOR OF THE EYEBALL

During the examination of the exterior of your eye, your doctor will check the surface of the eye as well as the eyelids, looking for potential problems such as redness, dryness, irritation, swelling, and microscopic scratches. He or she will also evaluate the movement of your eyes, both separately and together.

Your doctor will examine the exterior surface of the eyeball with a slit lamp, a table-mounted microscope that allows the doctor to see both the surface and the interior of the eyeball with amazing detail. For instance, the slit lamp allows the doctor to see tiny individual blood vessels in the retina that are less than one-tenth of a millimeter wide.

In general, problems that involve the exterior surface of the eye usually do not affect vision. They can, however, cause discomfort and affect the appearance of your eye. For instance, a scratch on the surface of your cornea will cause a sharp pain every time you blink. Engorged surface blood vessels in the conjunctiva may cause your eyes to appear red or bloodshot. Other symptoms such as mucus, tearing, swelling, sharp pain, scratchiness, itching, and generalized discomfort usually reflect problems with the exterior surface of the eyeball. Examples of common and annoying conditions that affect the eye's exterior include dry eyes, misdirected eyelashes, styes and other lid problems, and conjunctivitis (pink eye).

INTERIOR OF THE EYEBALL

It is during the examination of the interior of the eyeball that your doctor will determine whether you have a cataract. Prior to examining your eye interior, the doctor

will dilate your pupil with eye drops. Why is this important? The lens of the eye and other important structures
are located behind the iris and pupil. When light strikes
our pupils, they constrict, or become smaller, making it
difficult for the doctor to see inside the eyeball. The dilating drops temporarily inhibit this reaction. During the
examination, the doctor will also use several illuminat-
ing and magnifying instruments, including the slit lamp,
to examine the inside of your eyeball (see Figure 3-1).

If you have a cataract, the slit lamp also makes it possible for the doctor to determine the characteristics of
the cataract. Is the cataract diffuse, meaning the entire
lens is cloudy? Or is the cataract focal, with the cloudiness appearing in patches? To better understand how a
cataract may be forming, consider the analogy of dust
on a car windshield. A layer of dust may cover the entire
windshield, and it may be a light layer or quite thick,
or splotches of dirt may appear on various parts of the
windshield. Similarly, the cloudiness created by the cataract may take many shapes or forms.

While your pupil is dilated, the doctor will also check
those structures that lie behind the iris and the lens,
including the vitreous humor, retina, and optic nerve.
Abnormalities with any of these structures could create
vision problems.

When the pupil has been dilated, it allows more light
than usual to enter the eye. Therefore, you may feel
uncomfortable in bright environments while your eyes
are dilated. You may be more comfortable wearing sunglasses when you leave the doctor's office. The dilating
drops wear off in several hours.

MEASURING EYE PRESSURE

Another important part of the complete eye examination is the measurement of the eye's internal fluid pressure, or intraocular pressure. What is this fluid and why is the pressure important? It is a clear fluid called *aqueous humor* that circulates through the interior of the eyeball to keep it properly inflated.

As we age, the microscopic drainage area within the eye can clog. If fluid does not drain properly, pressure gradually increases. You can't feel this pressure; the amount of fluid is only about one-sixteenth teaspoon. However, over time the excessive fluid pressure can seriously damage the optic nerve. This condition is known as *glaucoma*. Once it is diagnosed, the high fluid pressure can be lowered with eye drop medications.

Measuring internal eye fluid pressure is safe, simple, and painless. The doctor uses anesthetic eye drops to numb the surface of the eyeball. He or she then uses a tonometer, a special pressure-sensing probe that is usually mounted on the slit lamp microscope, to determine the pressure in the eyeball.

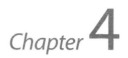

Your Intraocular Lens

T hanks to modern medicine, cataract treatment today involves an efficient surgical procedure during which the clouded lens is removed and a new, permanent, artificial lens is inserted into the eye. This lens is called an *intraocular lens*, or IOL. The development of the IOL was a remarkable achievement and represents one of the most important medical advances in the history of ophthalmology.

Invention of the IOL

Prior to the development of the IOL, patients had to wear extremely strong and thick eyeglasses following cataract surgery to replace the missing function of the extracted human lens. These extremely thick eyeglasses were heavy and produced magnified eyesight that was unnatural and difficult to adapt to. During the Second World War, British ophthalmologist Harold

Chang DF, Lee BS.
Cataracts: A Patient's Guide to Treatment,
Third Edition (pp 31-44).
© 2016 SLACK Incorporated.

Ridley treated several fighter pilots who had splinters from shattered aircraft canopies penetrating the interior of their eyeballs. To his amazement, Ridley found that, unlike other foreign materials that became lodged inside the eyeball following injuries, these pieces of plastic did not cause severe inflammation. He decided to see if a similar plastic could be used to make an artificial lens to replace the natural lens removed in cataract surgery.

In 1949, Ridley courageously performed the first IOL implant surgery. His lens design and surgical techniques were crude by today's standards, so his results weren't always satisfactory. Nevertheless, his work was a monumental event in the history of ophthalmology.

Like many visionaries, Ridley and his ideas were initially ridiculed by the medical establishment. Most doctors felt that it was too risky to insert objects permanently into the eye, and the idea of lens implantation was nearly abandoned.

Fortunately, research continued, and after nearly 20 years of experimentation with IOL designs by numerous surgeons in several countries, the modern IOL was developed (Table 4-1). Today's IOL brings no unwanted magnification and provides the most natural vision possible.

The development of the IOL represents one of the most important advances in the history of ophthalmology.

IOLs are permanent, require no handling or care, and come in a wide range of powers that are individually selected for each individual patient.

Manufacturing of IOLs

Modern IOLs are made of either silicone or acrylic plastic and are foldable. Folding the lens allows doctors

Table 4-1.
Characteristics of Modern IOLs
• Permanently fixed inside the eye • Made of a transparent material that does not cloud • No moving parts that can wear out • Lightweight and flexible • Not affected by physical activities or by rubbing the eye • Cannot be felt within the eye • Provide the best possible vision correction • Do not require cleaning • Do not change the appearance or comfort of the eye • Can be folded for insertion through a small incision, then unfolds to original size

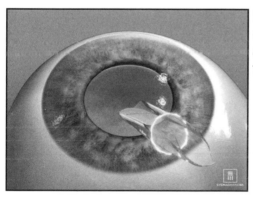

Figure 4-1. Foldable IOLs can be inserted through a small incision, leading to a faster recovery.

to implant it through a very small incision (Figure 4-1). Foldable IOLs are also associated with less frequent clouding of the supporting lens capsule that sits directly behind the artificial lens. Although they are more expensive to manufacture, foldable lenses are now the preferred lens implant in developed countries.

Figure 4-2. The artificial lens implant is permanently held and supported by the original lens capsule, which is preserved by the surgery.

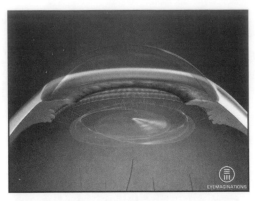

Figure 4-3. A posterior chamber IOL in the eye.

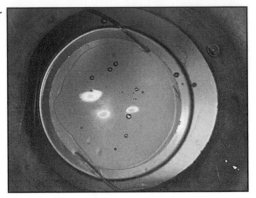

Placement of the IOL

When the IOL is placed in front of the iris, it is called an *anterior chamber IOL*. If it is placed in the capsular bag behind the iris, it is referred to as a *posterior chamber IOL*. There is no difference in optical quality, vision, or comfort between the 2 types of IOLs. The anterior chamber IOL was preferred in earlier years when cataract surgeons were limited to techniques that removed the entire lens with its support structures. As surgical techniques evolved, the capsular bag was able to be preserved for lens support, and the posterior chamber IOL became the preferred design (Figures 4-2 and 4-3).

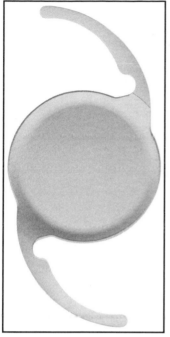

Figure 4-4. This is a monofocal IOL. (Reprinted with permission from Abbott Medical Optics.)

Types of IOLs

MONOFOCAL

Conventional IOLs are single-focus, or monofocal, lenses. They cannot change focus from far distance to near (Figure 4-4). Following cataract surgery, patients may be able to perform many activities without glasses, but patients will need to choose from the same options available to everyone else over the age of 50—contact lenses, bifocals, or separate driving or reading eyeglasses—to optimize their focus at different distances.

Nowadays, there are special "refractive" IOLs that can reduce (but generally not eliminate) your dependence on eyeglasses. The term *refractive* describes the fact that these designs provide no health or safety advantages,

Figure 4-5. This is a multifocal IOL. (Reproduced with permission of Alcon.)

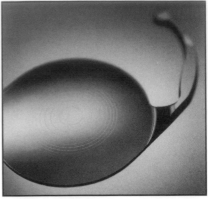

but rather offer the convenience of seeing better without eyeglasses. Because this convenience is not medically necessary, the additional costs for refractive IOLs are not covered by insurance and must be paid by the patient.

MULTIFOCAL IOLS

Multifocal IOLs are designed to produce a dual focus—part of the lens is set for distance focus and part of the lens is set for near focus (Figure 4-5). Therefore, compared to a monofocal lens implant set for distance focus only, a multifocal IOL should improve one's ability to see close up without glasses. Patients who receive a multifocal lens enjoy the convenience of requiring reading glasses much less often than with a conventional monofocal lens. However, they generally still wear reading glasses for some tasks, such as prolonged reading or close work.

PSEUDOACCOMMODATING IOLS

Pseudoaccommodating IOLs do not actually move or change shape inside the eye as the natural human lens does. However, they provide greater range and depth of focus than a conventional monofocal IOL (Figure 4-6). Although there is individual variability in how much

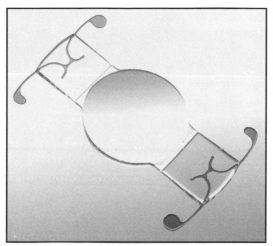

Figure 4-6. This is a pseudoaccommodating IOL. (Reprinted with permission from Bausch + Lomb.)

near vision they provide, pseudoaccommodating IOLs should reduce how often eyeglasses need to be worn in comparison to conventional monofocal lenses.

The advantages of both multifocal and pseudoaccommodating IOLs may be reduced, however, if there is too much astigmatism or if there are other eye problems.

TORIC IOLS

Toric IOLs are a type of monofocal lens implant used to correct astigmatism (Figure 4-7). Astigmatism, an imperfection in the natural shape of one's cornea, causes an undesirable blur or misfocus and can be corrected with prescription spectacles. By placing this optical correction directly into the toric IOL, the natural sight without glasses is better than with a conventional monofocal IOL for eyes with astigmatism.

The 3 categories of refractive IOLs (multifocal, pseudoaccommodating, and toric) are discussed in more detail in Chapter 8. Although refractive IOLs don't generally eliminate the need for eyeglasses, they are designed to

Figure 4-7. This is a toric IOL. Note the 2 sets of 3 dots, which are used to align the lens properly in order to correct the astigmatism from the cornea. (Reproduced with permission of Alcon.)

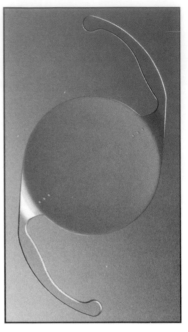

reduce how often patients require the use of their glasses by improving their natural vision without spectacles.

Selecting Your Lens Implant Power

At some point prior to your surgery, your doctor will need to determine the power of the IOL that will replace the optical power once provided by your natural lens. Regardless of whether it is a refractive or a conventional monofocal IOL, each model is available in more than 60 powers. The central viewing area of the IOL, which provides the optical power, is called the *optic*. This is a clear, round disc measuring about 6 millimeters in diameter (about one-fourth inch). As with other types of lenses, the optical power of IOLs is measured in units called *diopters*.

Your surgeon will select a specific lens power for your IOL with the goal of achieving your target focal distance. With your input, the surgeon must decide approximately where (far, near, or intermediate focus) to target your uncorrected vision (without glasses) after IOL surgery. Your lifestyle, the vision of your other eye, and your prior eyeglass prescription are all factors to consider. If, for instance, it's especially important for you to be able to read up close without glasses, you may prefer to remain nearsighted after cataract surgery.

Many patients want to see as well as possible in the distance without eyeglasses. For others, a slight amount of myopia (nearsightedness) may represent a good compromise between having very blurred vision for either far distance or near distance without glasses. Some people elect to have one eye be focused for distance vision without glasses and the other for closer vision—this is called *monovision* or *blended vision*. However, not everyone can comfortably adjust to this imbalance in focal distance.

Compounding the challenge of choosing a proper lens implant power is the fact that with IOLs you cannot try out different powers as you can when getting eyeglasses or contact lenses. Because the IOL is placed inside the eyeball after the natural lens has been removed, there is no way to preview different IOL powers in advance.

Instead, your surgeon will use a computer program to help estimate the appropriate IOL power before surgery. The computer calculations are based on the dimensions of your eyeball. Performed in the doctor's office, these painless measurements determine the amount of corneal curvature (which correlates with the cornea's optical power) and the distance from the cornea to the retina. Because this distance cannot be determined with a ruler, ultrasound technology was developed to measure this distance in tenths of a millimeter.

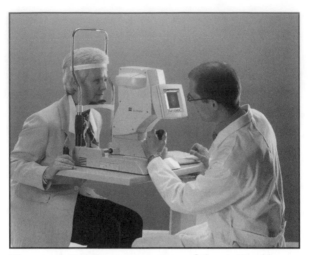

Figure 4-8. Measurements of the retinal location are painlessly performed with advanced scanning technology. This measurement is important for the determination of the optimal power of the IOL. (Reprinted with permission from Carl Zeiss Meditec.)

A more recent advance in IOL power selection has been the use of a scanning diagnostic laser beam to measure the precise location of the retina to within one-hundredth of a millimeter (Figure 4-8). Like existing ultrasound technology, this method is safe, painless, and fast and provides the most accurate measurement.

Another technology, called *intraoperative aberrometry*, is used by the surgeon in the operating room during the surgical procedure. This allows additional measurements of the eye's focusing power to be taken after the cataract has been removed. This machine is incorporated into the operating microscope. The additional information helps the surgeon with IOL power selection and may be particularly valuable in patients who have had prior refractive surgery such as LASIK or photorefractive keratectomy.

This intraoperative technology is usually not covered by insurance. It is discussed further in Chapters 8 and 9.

Finally, it is important to remember that even with refinements in taking measurements for IOL power, determining target focus and selecting the appropriate lens implant power is an imperfect process. For example, another factor affecting the outcome is the final resting position of the IOL inside the eyeball, which the doctor can only estimate prior to surgery. Still, eyeglasses can always be prescribed to provide excellent distance vision after cataract surgery and correct any lingering refractive error.

Secondary IOLs

Although it is uncommon, some patients may not have received an IOL at the time of their original cataract surgery. In these cases, an IOL can still be implanted many years later. This type of IOL is called a *secondary IOL implant* because it is inserted during a second operation. Several different designs can be used for secondary IOLs, depending upon where within the eye the IOL can be best supported. If enough of the lens capsule remains, it may support a posterior chamber IOL. If not, an anterior chamber IOL can be positioned in front of the iris. For some people, prior injuries or surgical complications may have resulted in internal iris scarring or defects that make it difficult to support an anterior chamber IOL. Even in these cases, posterior chamber IOLs can be permanently sutured into place.

If you need a secondary IOL, your surgeon will determine which design is optimal based upon your eye's specific anatomy.

Commonly Asked Questions About IOLs

How Long Have IOLs Been Used?

The first IOLs in North America were used in the early 1970s; however, at first only a few surgeons used them. The use of IOLs became prevalent in the early 1980s, and today they are used in all cataract operations.

How Long Will the IOL Last?

The IOL is permanent, and unlike an artificial joint or heart valve, there are no moving parts to wear out.

Even artificial lenses implanted in children following congenital cataract surgery are expected to last a lifetime.

Can the IOL Be Removed and Replaced?

Although it is rarely necessary, the IOL can be removed and replaced. One reason for replacement would be that, despite all of the preliminary calculations, the power is incorrect. Eyes that have undergone a prior LASIK or radial keratotomy procedure are at greater risk for this problem. Another reason would be if the IOL shifted out of position inside the eye, a very rare event. Because the artificial lens is designed to be permanent, removing it is generally not a simple task.

Does the IOL Replace the Need for Sunglasses?

Sunglasses provide 2 benefits: their darker tint reduces the brightness of our surroundings by decreasing the amount of light that reaches the eye, and the major health benefit is that they contain a transparent coating that blocks the ultraviolet (UV) rays of the sun. UV rays are what cause sunburn, and they are present even on overcast days. Because of the potential for cumulative damage to the retina, it is advisable to block out UV light. All modern IOLs permanently provide this UV protection at all times. Because IOLs have no dark tinting, patients may still choose to wear sunglasses for comfort, just as they did before their cataract surgery.

WHERE ARE IOLS MANUFACTURED?

Although IOLs are manufactured in many industrialized countries, the IOLs commonly used in North America are produced in the United States. The quality control is very strict and must be of the highest standard to obtain the United States Food and Drug Administration's (FDA) approval. In the developing world, inexpensive IOLs may be produced locally; these are not subject to the rigid standards of the FDA.

HOW IS THE IOL PAID FOR?

In most surgical facilities, the cost of a conventional monofocal, foldable IOL is either absorbed into a single flat fee for the operation, or it is part of a cost allowance determined by the insurer, such as Medicare. As mentioned earlier, patients may elect to pay the additional costs to receive a refractive IOL to improve their ability to see without eyeglasses.

Summary

You can enjoy the benefits of current IOL designs that have evolved over the past 3 decades and have a proven track record after being implanted in millions of eyes annually. Rest assured that all of the IOLs used in North America have passed rigorous long-term testing for optical quality, safety, and performance. Current IOL manufacturing in the United States is done under strict quality controls and meets the highest possible industry standards.

Figures 4-1 and 4-2 have been reprinted with permission from Eyemaginations.

Chapter 5

Planning for Cataract Surgery

Being diagnosed with cataracts can produce feelings of anxiety. Understandably, anything that goes wrong with our eyes can feel scary. Fortunately, vision problems caused by cataracts are reversible. Today, cataract removal is one of the most common and successful surgeries done in the United States, with more than 3 million procedures performed annually. The number is expected to grow as the population ages.

If you have cataracts that are causing vision problems, you and your ophthalmologist will need to decide when it's time to remove them. Once cataracts form, there are no medications, eye drops, exercises, glasses, supplements, or herbs that can cause them to disappear. Cataracts must be removed through a surgical procedure, and a new, artificial lens implant—the intraocular lens— must be inserted to restore vision.

Chang DF, Lee BS.
*Cataracts: A Patient's Guide to Treatment,
Third Edition* (pp 45-54).
© 2016 SLACK Incorporated.

The good news is that, once removed, a cataract will never come back. And you're never too old to have cataract surgery because you're never too old to enjoy the benefits of better vision. Unfortunately, some people try to adapt to poorer vision, accepting it as a normal part of aging. However, they often do not realize how poor their vision has actually become, nor do they realize how much their vision could be improved with cataract surgery.

When Should Cataracts Be Removed?

You should consider having a cataract operation when cataract removal will noticeably improve your vision.

You should consider having a cataract operation when cataract removal will noticeably improve your vision. Cataracts progress at surprisingly different rates. Some cataracts hardly seem to change for years, and others progress quickly. It is virtually impossible for your doctor to predict how quickly an early cataract will progress. As cataracts inevitably worsen, the need for surgery becomes more obvious over time.

Your lifestyle and occupational needs should be central to your decision. For example, if your job or hobby requires excellent eyesight, you might elect to have surgery much earlier than someone who doesn't have the same vision requirements. You'll also want to consider the rate at which your vision is declining. Most cataracts eventually advance to a point at which the worsening accelerates more and more rapidly. Talk with your eye doctor about how your cataracts are affecting your vision and your life. Although your doctor cannot make the final decision for you, he or she can help you weigh the pros and cons.

Here are some questions you might ask your doctor:

- Would new eyeglasses improve my vision?
- Would I be able to pass a driving test right now?
- Is my cataract mild, medium, or advanced?
- Would the improvement from cataract surgery be subtle or obvious?
- Do I have any other problems besides cataracts that are reducing my vision?
- Does my eye pose any special problems or risks for cataract surgery?
- What restrictions will I have following surgery?
- If I have surgery, how long will I be out of work?
- If I currently need strong prescription glasses to see, what will my prescription be like following surgery?
- Is surgery covered by my insurance? If not, how much will it cost?

Having a cataract diagnosed doesn't mean you have to have it removed immediately. Most people have plenty of time to decide when to have cataract surgery. You and your doctor can decide when to have your cataracts removed based on how much the cataract is impairing your vision.

Benefits of Cataract Surgery

- Improved eyesight (Figure CA-2)
- Improved color vision and night vision
- Improved functional abilities for reading, driving, and occupational tasks
- Depending on the lens implant, decreased dependence on eyeglasses

- For those with large preoperative refractive errors, an improvement in their eyeglass prescription
- Less frequent need to change eyeglasses in the future
- A permanent end to the progressive worsening in vision caused by cataracts

Who Performs Cataract Surgery?

Ophthalmologists perform cataract surgery, and you'll want an ophthalmologist who is experienced. Good cataract surgeons are much like good golfers—they are trained well and develop their skills through much practice. Based on years of experience, they are prepared for almost any situation and can perform well under pressure. As with any high-level skill, the more a professional practices, the better he or she will be. As you'd expect, ophthalmologists who perform a greater number of cataract surgeries are more likely to have the most current and well-honed skills.

Finding the Right Cataract Surgeon

If your cataracts have been diagnosed and followed by an optometrist or an ophthalmologist who doesn't perform cataract surgery, you will need a referral to a cataract surgeon when you are ready for surgery. Your current eye doctor will usually be able to recommend a good cataract surgeon for you. After receiving the recommendation, ask your eye doctor if he or she has cared for others who have had their cataracts removed by that surgeon. You also can ask friends, family, coworkers, and other physicians for recommendations.

Check to see that your ophthalmologist is board certified. This means he or she has passed a rigorous examination given by a board of peers. Take the time to learn about his or her credentials through the doctor's office brochure or website.

When you meet with the surgeon, it is important that he or she makes you feel comfortable. You should be able to ask questions and have them answered in a manner that you understand. Becoming knowledgeable about cataracts, gaining confidence in your surgeon, and maintaining a positive attitude about your condition can help make your cataract surgery experience much easier.

How a Cataract Is Removed

The preferred technique for cataract removal is called *extracapsular surgery*, but there are 2 different ways to do it: a small-incision or a large-incision method. In both methods, the surgeon makes a circular incision in the front of the capsular bag, the outer covering of the lens. As you may recall from the earlier discussion of eye anatomy, the capsule is a thin, transparent covering that encases the natural lens like a delicate cellophane wrapper. During extracapsular surgery, the back half of the capsular bag is left intact when the cloudy lens is removed. This provides a supporting sac-like structure to hold the artificial lens implant.

SMALL-INCISION SURGERY

The most common extracapsular surgical technique in North America is small-incision surgery (Table 5-1). Virtually all ophthalmologists use this technique. As the name implies, only a small incision, measuring approximately 3 millimeters (about one-eighth inch), is required (Figure 5-1).

Once the incision is made, the cataract is removed with an instrument called a *phacoemulsifier*. This instrument

Table 5-1.
Advantages of Small-Incision Cataract Surgery
• Surgery can be performed more quickly
• Topical anesthesia (using eye drops) can be used instead of local-injection anesthesia
• It is safer if a patient accidentally moves or coughs during surgery
• No routine need for sutures
• Faster healing of the incision
• Generally no need to restrict exercise or physical activity
• Quicker recovery of sight
• New eyeglasses can be prescribed much sooner
• Less risk of the procedure creating or worsening astigmatism
• Permits the use of the newer, foldable intraocular lenses
• Less frequent need to change eyeglasses in the future

was originally designed in the 1970s but has since undergone continuous improvement, especially with modern computer technology. Once inserted, the microscopic phacoemulsifier probe uses ultrasound waves vibrating at 40,000 times per second to break up the cloudy lens gently (Figure CA-5). This process is called *phacoemulsification*, or *phaco* for short. The pieces of lens are carefully vacuumed out, and the new, foldable intraocular lens is inserted into the empty capsular bag, where it opens to its full size (Figures 5-2 through 5-4, Figure CA-6). Over a period of several weeks, the capsular bag contracts, essentially shrinkwrapping the lens implant and holding it firmly in place (Figure CA-7).

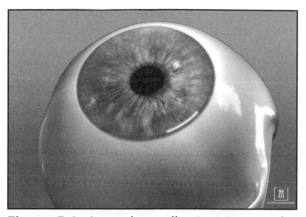

Figure 5-1. A much smaller incision can be used if the cataract is fragmented ultrasonically. Frequently, no stitches are required because outward pressure from fluid within the eyeball seals the incision.

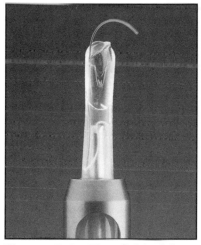

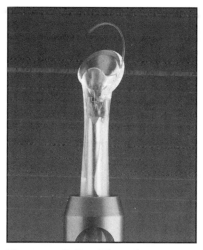

Figure 5-2. The folded lens can be inserted through a tiny incision by using this special injector system. (Reprinted with permission from Abbott Medical Optics.)

Figure 5-3. The lens can be carefully positioned as it slowly emerges from the injector tip. (Reprinted with permission from Abbott Medical Optics.)

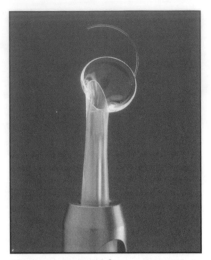

Figure 5-4. After emerging into the eye, the artificial lens unfolds to its regular shape. (Reprinted with permission from Abbott Medical Optics.)

Sutures are usually not required because the tiny incision is fashioned into a flap that closes on its own. Because the incision is so small, actions such as coughing, straining, or inadvertently rubbing the eye are not harmful. Accordingly, physical activities are not restricted after small-incision surgery.

LARGE-INCISION SURGERY

The large-incision method was the most popular extracapsular cataract procedure prior to the 1990s. In large-incision surgery, the solid central core of the cataract, called the *nucleus*, is removed intact rather than being broken apart by phaco. The nucleus makes up 90% of the volume of the lens, requiring a larger incision to remove it in one piece. The incision for this procedure is up to 12 millimeters long (one-half inch), compared to

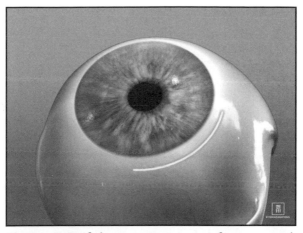

Figure 5-5. If the cataract is not fragmented, a larger incision is needed to extract the solid portion. This large incision must be closed with multiple stitches and is no longer the preferred method.

one-eighth inch for small-incision surgery (Figure 5-5). Closing the large incision might require 8 or 9 sutures. Some doctors who are not experienced in small-incision surgery may still use this method. Occasionally, a patient is a poor candidate for small-incision surgery; the cataract may be too dense to remove with ultrasound, or the capsular bag may be too weak to allow phaco. These patients can have large-incision extracapsular cataract surgery and do well.

Because a large-incision procedure weakens the wall of the eye, a patient must limit physical activity for up to 4 weeks. Even bending over to tie a shoelace can strain the incision, and exercise must often be significantly restricted.

The large-incision procedure also causes greater changes in the shape of the cornea, which usually increases astigmatism. Tight sutures may cause excessive astigmatism that requires cutting the offending sutures after 6 weeks. For this reason, people might receive a temporary eyeglass prescription initially and a final eyeglass prescription several months later. To protect the eye from injury and to prevent rupturing the sutures by accidental rubbing, a patient wears a metal guard over the eye while sleeping.

Figures 5-1 and 5-5 have been reprinted with permission from Eyemaginations.

Color Atlas

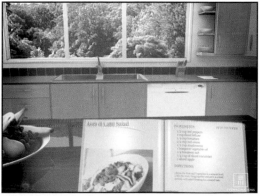

Figure CA-1. Some cataracts still permit patients to read and see details but cause a haziness to the vision.

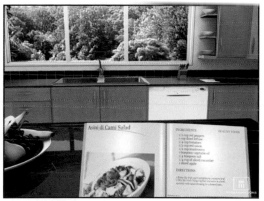

Figure CA-2. Cataract surgery improves the quality and clarity of vision.

Cataract Surgery Steps

Figure CA-3. A small incision is made at the edge of the cornea.

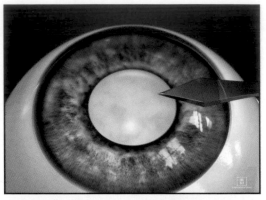

Figure CA-4. A circular opening in the front of the lens capsule is made to gain access to the cataract.

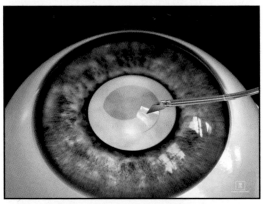

Figure CA-5. The cataract is fragment- ed and emulsified with a microscopic instrument called the *phaco tip.*

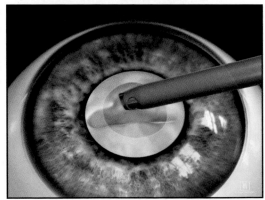

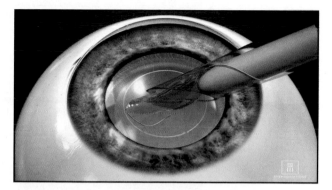

Figure CA-6. Foldable lens implants can be inserted through much smaller incisions.

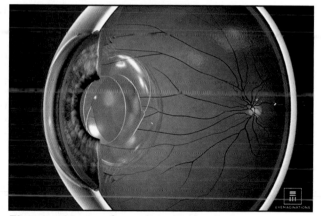

Figure CA-7. After the artificial lens implant unfolds, it is permanently held inside the original capsular bag that surrounded the human lens. By using this same support structure from the human lens, it is not necessary to clip or stitch the lens implant to hold it in place.

YAG Laser Treatment

Figure CA-8. A secondary membrane refers to clouding of the back portion of the lens capsule, which sits directly behind the artificial lens implant. Shown as a grayish-white haze in this picture, this clouding of the formerly transparent capsule causes the vision to become blurry or hazy.

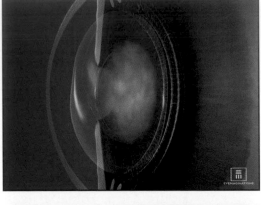

Figure CA-9. A laser beam is used to make a small permanent hole in the center of the back capsule. The microscopic precision of the laser allows it to make this opening in the capsule without damaging the artificial lens implant in front of it.

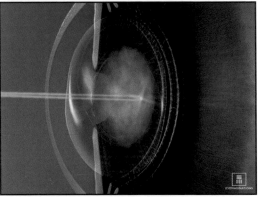

Figure CA-10. Like a window, this permanent opening restores clear vision through the eye's visual axis. The remainder of the capsular bag is unaffected and continues to support the artificial lens implant.

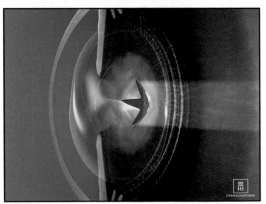

Chapter 6

Undergoing
Cataract Surgery

Not so long ago, cataract surgery involved an overnight stay in the hospital. Today, cataract surgery is performed on an outpatient basis. The procedure is usually done in an ambulatory surgery center or in the outpatient department of a hospital. Some cataract surgeons have surgical facilities adjoining their offices. Because they are surgical procedures, cataract operations should be performed in fully equipped operating rooms under antiseptic conditions to minimize the risk of infection.

Once you arrive at the surgery center, several steps will be taken to prepare you for your cataract removal. Although the surgery itself takes less than half an hour, because of the preoperative preparations and paperwork involved, you'll likely spend several hours at the surgery center.

Chang DF, Lee BS.
Cataracts: A Patient's Guide to Treatment,
Third Edition (pp 55-67).
© 2016 SLACK Incorporated.

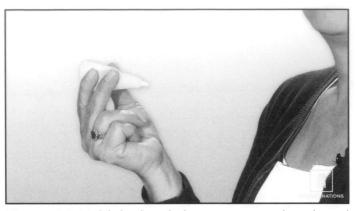

Figure 6-1. Hold the bottle between your thumb and your index and middle fingers of your right hand (if right handed).

Prior to Surgery

USING EYE DROP MEDICATIONS

One or more days prior to surgery, you may be asked to use antibiotic eye drops, and your eye doctor will instruct you in their use (Figures 6-1 through 6-4). The drops are intended to kill any bacteria that could cause an infection. Properly using prescribed eye drop medications before and after surgery is important to the success of your cataract surgery. If you've never used eye drops, it may take just a bit of practice to get them into your eye; the natural reflex is to blink to avoid the drops. But it shouldn't take you long to learn how to use them properly.

The goal is to have the drop land anywhere on the exterior surface of the eyeball. The medication will spread across the eyeball's surface, and within a few minutes, it will penetrate the cornea to the eye's interior.

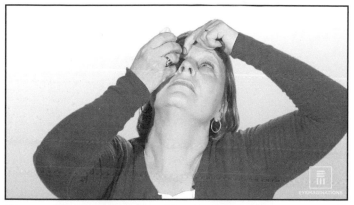

Figure 6-2. Tip your head back. Next, place your right pinky on your cheek to steady your hand as you position the inverted bottle tip over the eye. Use one of your left fingers to lift the upper eyelid.

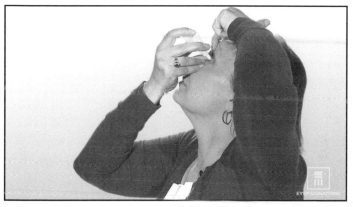

Figure 6-3. The fourth and fifth fingers of the right hand can pull the lower lid down. By retracting the lower lid with the right hand and the upper lid with the left hand, you are widening the space between the upper and lower eyelids. This is the target area for the eye drop to land—on the eye surface between the upper and lower eyelid/eyelash margins.

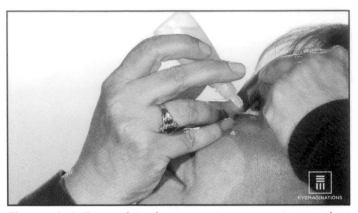

Figure 6-4. From this close-up view, you can see that the eye drop tip should not touch the eye surface.

It is important to close your eye and not to blink too much after putting in eye drops. Blinking pumps the eye drop medication off the eye surface toward the openings of the tear ducts. To reduce blinking, gently close the eye without squeezing the eyelid for at least 1 minute after putting in the drop.

The eye drop will be effective if it lands on either the eyeball or on the pinkish inside surface of the lower eyelid. However, if the eye drop lands on the eyelid skin or on the lashes, you'll have to try again. Whenever possible, it is recommended to wash your hands before using eye drops. Eye drop instillation is easiest if you either lie down or tilt your head back (Figure 6-5).

You need only one drop of medication for one dose. Don't worry if you accidentally apply several drops; it won't harm the eye. If you think you missed your eye, it's okay to apply another drop. For more than one type of eye drop medication, allow 3 minutes or more between each type of medication so that the first drop is not immediately rinsed out by the second.

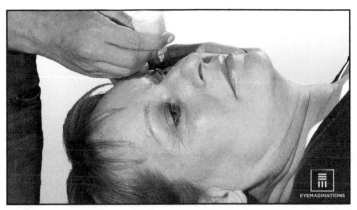

Figure 6-5. Lying down can also help, particularly if someone is assisting you.

While you're first learning to use eye drops, you may want to refrigerate your eye drops. It makes it easier to tell whether the drop lands on the eyeball. Some people rely on a spouse or other family member to help them with eye drops. Even if you have this option, it's better if you learn to do it for yourself in case your helper isn't available.

OTHER MEDICATIONS

Continue taking your regular medications, such as blood pressure medication, unless your surgeon tells you otherwise. Many ophthalmologists even allow their patients to continue taking aspirin and other blood thinners because the risk of serious bleeding with small-incision cataract surgery and topical anesthesia is extremely low.

FOOD AND DRINK

Depending on the time of your scheduled surgery, your doctor may ask you not to eat or drink anything on the morning of your surgery. If so, you might wish to have a snack before going to bed the night before so you don't feel too hungry. If you're diabetic and take insulin or pill medications, your doctor may ask you to reduce or skip your morning dose before surgery.

BEFORE LEAVING HOME

Here are some important things to be aware of before heading to the surgery center:

- Make sure you have your insurance cards and related information. Some surgery centers may request that you complete a brief health question-naire.
- Know who is going to drive you home. Because you'll be receiving mild sedation during surgery, this arrangement is necessary. If you don't have a family member or friend who can drive you home, ask your ophthalmologist's staff about possible alternatives.
- Wear loose, comfortable clothing.
- Do not apply makeup.
- Leave jewelry and valuables at home.
- If you take nitroglycerin pills or use inhalers for asthma or other breathing problems, take them along.

Preoperative Preparations

In the preoperative area, you'll be asked to sit in a chair or lie on a bed. If you have any problems lying flat, be sure to tell the nurse so the bed can be adjusted to make you comfortable. During this presurgery period, a friend or family member may usually keep you company.

A nurse will measure your vital signs, blood pressure, and heart rate. To help you relax, you'll probably be given a mild anti-anxiety medication. An intravenous (IV) line may be started in your arm or hand so that sedative medication can be administered during surgery as needed. The goal of the sedation is to help you relax but not fall asleep during the surgery. It might make you quite drowsy, and patients often do not remember parts of the procedure.

The nursing staff will administer eye drop medications into the eye undergoing the procedure. Some surgery centers use either a gel or a tiny, soft sponge called a *pledget* to administer eye medications. The nurse will gently place the gel or sponge under the eyelid in the corner where it won't bother you. One medication will be dilating drops that are similar to those used in routine eye examinations. Because of the strength of these eye drops, your pupil may still be dilated the next day.

Some people doze off during this preoperative period. Others bring a portable music player and headphones to pass the time.

Receiving Anesthesia

Cataract surgery is generally associated with minimal discomfort. Two types of anesthesia, both local, are commonly used for the procedure. Many doctors use topical anesthesia eye drops. Other doctors use regional anesthesia, which is administered by injection. The choice of anesthesia will depend on your surgeon's preference. Both types numb the eyeball well.

In years past, regional anesthesia, a longer-acting anesthesia delivered by injection, was the most commonly used anesthetic for cataract surgery. Today, topical anesthesia is the preference of many surgeons. Topical anesthesia, however, can be used only with small-incision surgery.

Only in special cases would a doctor use general anesthesia, which puts the patient to sleep. For example, general anesthesia may be used for patients who can't cooperate, such as children or adults with advanced dementia.

REGIONAL ANESTHESIA

If you are having a regional anesthetic, your doctor will inject Novocain (procaine) or a similar agent into your lower eyelid. This numbs the eyeball by anesthetizing the nerves leading to it. After the surgery, the eye must be patched or taped shut until the anesthetic wears off. Why an eye patch? The longer-acting anesthetic injection temporarily weakens the muscles that control blinking, the eye's defense mechanism against drying and having something touch its surface. For this reason, the eye must be kept closed until the anesthetic agents wear off, which can take many hours. For many patients, the patch will be removed the following morning.

TOPICAL ANESTHESIA

If you are undergoing topical anesthesia, the doctor will administer anesthetic eye drops. Patients usually require less sedation during surgery when they receive anesthesia in this way. Another advantage to topical anesthesia is that it prevents potential side effects from the needle injection, such as discomfort, bruising, swelling, or temporary drooping of the eyelids. And because the topical medication does not affect the surrounding muscles, no eye bandage is required at the end of the surgery.

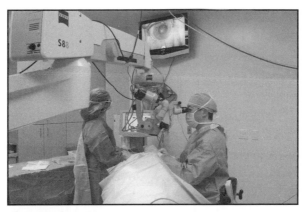

Figure 6-6. Eye surgeons use an operating microscope to perform cataract surgery.

Undergoing Small-Incision Cataract Removal

Before your procedure, the nurse will cleanse the skin around your eye and cover your eyelids with a sterile plastic drape. Once the surgeon begins the operation, he or she will use a device called a *speculum* to gently hold the eyelids open so you cannot blink. You will be able to see light but not the instruments being used. In fact, patients commonly report that they see a kaleidoscope of beautiful colors and radiating light patterns during their operation. Patients are also aware of a cool, wet sensation as eye drops are used to rinse and moisten the eye's surface throughout the surgery. Although few patients report discomfort, many say they feel pressure on their eyeball at times during the procedure.

With the help of a high-powered operating microscope, the surgeon performs cataract surgery inside the eye (Figure 6-6). The following steps are involved in a small-incision procedure:

- A small incision in the cornea is made with an ultra-thin blade (Figure CA-3).
- A circular opening is made in front of the lens capsule (Figure CA-4).
- The tip of the phacoemulsification instrument is inserted through the incision into the opened capsular bag.
- The instrument gently breaks up the cloudy lens. The pieces are carefully suctioned from the eyeball (Figure CA-5).
- The intraocular lens is folded and inserted through the incision. The new lens unfolds to its permanent shape and is positioned inside the vacant capsular bag (Figures CA-6 and CA-7).
- The incision, fashioned as a flap valve, closes on its own. Typically, no sutures are needed.
- Special saline solution is administered to re-establish proper pressure inside the eyeball.

You'll be able to talk to the surgeon during the operation. For example, if you need to cough or sneeze, you can tell the doctor so he or she can stop momentarily. Many patients remark about how quickly the actual surgical procedure is performed.

After Your Surgery

After the procedure, you'll be taken to a recovery room where you'll rest briefly. The length of time needed to remain at the surgery center varies for each individual. Many patients are ready to be driven home within 15 minutes.

Before you return home, a nurse will check your pulse and blood pressure once more and review the immediate postoperative instructions with you. Because the sedative often makes it hard to remember details, many doctors send you home with written instructions. Because of the sedative, you should reread any written instructions on the day following surgery.

With small-incision surgery, you'll find you have few restrictions following surgery. If you've undergone topical anesthesia, you generally won't require an eye bandage. Because your eye was dilated during surgery, you will probably be more comfortable wearing sunglasses outdoors. The pupil will often remain dilated until the following day.

> *With small-incision surgery, you'll find you have few restrictions following surgery.*

In most cases, you will have a follow-up visit with your surgeon within the first 24 hours, or certainly within the next few days. During the follow-up visit, your sedative will have worn off, and you will likely feel more clearheaded. This will be a better time to ask questions about any long-term concerns you have.

Potential Risks

For most people, the chance of successful cataract surgery is greater than 98%. As with any operation, complications are possible, but severe complications that can cause permanent vision loss are rare. For example, the chance of major internal bleeding is less than 1 in 1000. The risk of infection is less than 1 in 1000.

Rare and unpredictable complications can occur with local or general anesthesia. Other uncommon, but possible, complications include the following:

- Prolonged elevation of intraocular pressure
- Persistent internal eye inflammation called *iritis*

- Macular edema (swelling) caused by microscopic amounts of fluid pooling in the center of the retina
- Corneal clouding caused by the depletion of cells that keep the cornea clear
- Problems with the retina, such as retinal detachment

Complications such as elevated pressure, iritis, and macular edema are treatable with eye drop medications. Permanent corneal clouding and retinal detachment are rare complications but possible risks if you are prone to these 2 complications. If they should occur, both are treated with surgery. If you are concerned about complications, discuss them with your eye surgeon.

Call your ophthalmologist immediately if you experience any of the following symptoms after surgery:

- Severe pain not relieved by nonprescription pain medication
- Sudden loss of vision
- Injury to the eye

Treatment for Cataracts in Both Eyes

If you have cataracts in both eyes, your cataract surgery will usually be performed on one eye at a time on different days. Your doctor wants to avoid your temporarily having blurred vision in both eyes during the healing process. Waiting also lets the surgeon assess the intraocular lens power chosen for the first procedure.

How soon can you have surgery in the second eye? It depends on how quickly your first eye recovers. Typically, cataract removal in the second eye takes place a few weeks after the first operation. Under certain circumstances, however, it may be possible for a person to undergo both operations within the same week. For example, if someone travels from out of town for the surgery, the second procedure might be scheduled within the same week to accommodate the patient.

Figures 6-1 through 6-5 have been reprinted with permission from Eyemaginations.

Chapter 7

Recovering From Surgery

Y our cataract surgery is over. You are the recipient of a new artificial lens, one of the amazing accomplishments of modern medicine! Your cataract will never come back, and your new intraocular lens (IOL) will never cloud.

If you are like the majority of individuals, you probably found that the entire cataract surgery experience was quicker and much easier than you expected. Over the next few days, your eyeball will be healing.

Returning to See Your Doctor

You'll probably have an appointment to see your eye surgeon at his or her office within 24 hours of your operation. This visit allows the doctor to check the incision, the condition of

Many people needlessly worry because they aren't seeing well immediately after surgery.

Chang DF, Lee BS.
*Cataracts: A Patient's Guide to Treatment,
Third Edition* (pp 69-80).
© 2016 SLACK Incorporated.

your eye, and its intraocular pressure. The doctor will also explain how often and how long you need to use postsurgical eye drop medications. This is also a good opportunity for you to ask any questions you might have.

Your doctor will conduct only a very limited vision test during this first visit after surgery. Naturally, you'll be curious about the results of your cataract surgery. However, many people needlessly worry because they aren't seeing well immediately after surgery. Blurred vision and other temporary postsurgical effects are common during recovery. They neither predict nor correlate with how well you'll see after your eye has healed.

Common Symptoms After Surgery

Immediately following your cataract surgery, you may experience a number of the following symptoms, which are normal and will disappear over time:

- Blurred and fluctuating vision
- Sensitivity to bright light
- Dilated pupil for 1 or 2 days
- Watery eyes
- Scratchy, sandy feeling in your eye
- Eye redness
- Stinging from eye drops
- Halos around lights at night
- Floaters
- Flickering vision or a curved dark shadow off to the side

If you find you are sensitive to light, sunglasses may make you feel more comfortable. However, because your new, artificial lens blocks out ultraviolet light, it is not medically necessary to wear sunglasses for ultraviolet protection.

Causes of Temporary Blurred Vision

At first, your vision will probably be quite blurred. If you underwent large-incision cataract surgery, your blurry vision might persist for several weeks. However, if you underwent small-incision cataract surgery and are like most people, you should notice your vision improving within a few days after your surgery. Keep in mind that these side effects are temporary. There are several reasons for the temporarily blurred vision.

DILATION OF THE PUPIL

Immediately after your surgery, your pupil will still be dilated. The effects of these drops may linger for more than 24 hours and may cause you to see an assortment of reflections and halos.

Patients sometimes describe seeing a "curved dark shadow off to the side." When the light enters at just the right angle, it is deflected by the edge of the IOL, and you see a momentary crescent-shaped shadow or shimmering of light. If you experience this side effect, be assured that it's normal and is a result of the IOL design. Although it may be distracting at first, you'll notice these curved shadows less and less over time. Also, after several months, the remaining capsule holding the IOL tends to cloud slightly around the implant's edge, which acts to significantly reduce these reflections.

MISTING OF THE CORNEA

Misting of the cornea is caused by microscopic swelling, which is a normal response to surgery. This misting, which may last for several days, creates temporary blurring. This reaction varies greatly among individuals. It will usually clear up during the first week.

MICROSCOPIC MOVEMENT OF THE IOL

After cataract surgery, some people notice a shimmering effect when they move their eyes. For example, at night when they look at car headlights or streetlights, they might see what appears to be a slight movement of the lighted object. This occurs as a result of a slight movement of the IOL. As you recall, during surgery, the IOL is placed inside the empty capsular bag. During the first week, the bag will contract and tighten around the artificial lens like a cellophane shrinkwrap. Until this happens, some slight jiggling movement of the IOL is normal. As a result of these slight movements, the eye's focus can vary during the first several days following surgery.

WRINKLE IN THE CAPSULAR BAG

You may notice starburst reflections at night as a result of a tiny wrinkle in the back portion of the capsular bag that holds your IOL. As the capsular bag starts to shrink and contract around the implanted IOL, this light-scattering wrinkle will usually smooth out and disappear.

Recovery After Surgery

After surgery, your doctor will have given you thorough instructions for caring for your eye during the healing phase. Whether your doctor restricts your activities depends on whether it was small- or large-incision surgery.

AFTER SMALL-INCISION SURGERY

It is more likely that you had small-incision cataract surgery. If so, you will have virtually no restrictions because the tiny incision does not weaken the wall of the eyeball. Although you should follow your surgeon's specific instructions, you can generally resume your everyday activities right away. You can also resume physical exercise such as golfing, jogging, or aerobics as soon as you wish. You don't have to worry about injury to your eye when you bend, stoop, lift, cough, or strain. You can read, use your computer, or watch television as much as you want. Soap and water won't harm your eye, so you don't have to worry about showering, washing your face or hair, or wearing makeup. You don't have to change your diet or alter your sleeping position. You can drive and return to work whenever you feel ready.

AFTER LARGE-INCISION SURGERY

If you had the less common large-incision surgery, you'll have restrictions in movement and physical activity. You will need to avoid heavy lifting, bending, and straining for several weeks following surgery. Such activities increase blood flow to the head, which exerts external pressure against the eyeball and the incision.

You'll need to wear an eye patch immediately after surgery and a protective metal eye shield at night for a few weeks. Your doctor may ask you to avoid getting water in the eye at first. Such guidelines will vary among doctors.

Using Eye Drops After Surgery

After your surgery, you will have been given a schedule for using eye drops. Anti-inflammatory eye drops will help decrease discomfort and light sensitivity and will speed healing. Antibiotic drops help prevent infection. These postoperative medications are usually continued for several weeks, and your doctor will give you instructions on when to taper or eliminate their use. Note that it is common for the drops to cause some stinging, especially on the first day or two.

If you wish, you can also take ibuprofen, Tylenol (acetaminophen), or other over-the-counter pain relievers to help with any postoperative aching that isn't relieved by eye drops or by taking a nap. In most cases, your eye will feel much better by the next morning.

USING MULTIPLE DROPS

You will likely be using several different kinds of eye drop medications. You can administer them in any order—just make sure you allow 3 minutes or more between each medication. This way, the second drop won't rinse away the first one before it has had time to be absorbed.

Frequently, when they reduce or stop using the post-surgery eye drops, patients may begin to notice some scratchiness or mild irritation. This suggests a tendency toward "dry eye," a common and harmless condition that's much like dry mouth or dry skin. If you have this symptom, using over-the-counter lubricant drops called *artificial tears* can help to reduce the irritation. You can use artificial tears anytime, but it is preferable to use preservative-free artificial tears if you are using them more than 3 times a day. Because of the microscopic cataract incision, the eye surface is more comfortable when it is well lubricated during the first several months following surgery. Most patients should consider using artificial tears at the first sign of any new irritation beyond the first few weeks.

Don't Compare Your Recovery to Others'

Don't worry if your postsurgery experience, including restrictions on activities following surgery, is different from that of others you know who have undergone cataract surgery. They may have undergone a different surgical technique, or their doctor may have a different postoperative routine. Comparing experiences can lead to considerable confusion. Following your surgeon's aftercare instructions, rather than the advice of friends and family, is your best bet.

Also, don't be concerned if your cataract surgery recovery rate is different from someone else's. Everyone heals at a different rate. Your recovery rate is normal for you. Many people even find differences in how they recovered from cataract surgery in each of their own 2 eyes. This is a frequent cause of unnecessary concern.

Wearing Your Eyeglasses After Surgery

Right after your cataract surgery, if your distance vision without glasses is good, you'll probably find you can't read well without glasses. While you wait for your new glasses, you might be able to wear an old pair of glasses for reading, or you may find that wearing over-the-counter reading glasses works. These inexpensive reading glasses are sold in most grocery and drug stores. They come in multiple standard powers ranging from +1.00 to +3.00 diopters and are available in half or full spectacle frames.

If you want to try these standard over-the-counter reading glasses but you're unsure what power to buy, simply try them on in the store to see which strength works best for you. Although these reading glasses will not work that well if your 2 eyes have different prescriptions and they will not correct astigmatism, many people find that they provide a functional and inexpensive option until new reading glasses can be prescribed.

When Will New Eyeglasses Be Prescribed?

Shortly after cataract surgery, your eyeglass prescription will change. After small-incision surgery, your prescription will stabilize much faster than after large-incision surgery. You can usually have your new glasses prescribed within several weeks of surgery. If you order them too soon, you may need to have them revised. If you're having cataracts removed from both eyes, it's generally a good idea to wait until after the second operation to change your eyeglass prescription. You won't, of course, be able to fully evaluate your true distance and near vision capabilities until you have your new eyeglasses.

Commonly Asked Questions About Recovery

WHEN CAN I DRIVE AGAIN?

There is no standard answer. Patients must decide for themselves at what point they see well enough to resume driving. Many patients are comfortable driving to their first postoperative visit on the morning after surgery. This is because surgery was performed on their worse eye, leaving the better eye unaffected. Obviously, if you feel your vision is not adequate, then don't drive.

HOW SOON CAN I TAKE THE EYE TEST FOR MY DRIVER'S LICENSE?

Although some patients will be able to pass the eye test without glasses, it is best to wait until the final postoperative refraction and vision test is administered several weeks following surgery. This way, if new corrective lenses are prescribed, you will have them available for taking the test. Understanding this, your local Department of Motor Vehicles will usually grant an extension.

IF I HAVE CATARACT SURGERY AND AN IOL IS INSERTED, CAN I WEAR CONTACTS?

Yes. In fact, if you want to use the strategy of monovision (one eye set for far focus and one eye set for near focus) to avoid glasses, it is often better to accomplish this with contact lenses. This way, the different focal points can be more precisely adjusted, and this state of disparate vision is reversible, in case it later becomes a disadvantage.

HOW SOON CAN I WEAR CONTACTS AFTER SURGERY?

Any previous contact lens will now have the wrong prescription. It is usually better to wait about 1 month after surgery before a new contact lens is prescribed and fitted.

I DON'T LIKE BIFOCALS. DO I HAVE TO HAVE THEM IN MY NEW EYEGLASSES?

As they are for everyone over the age of 45, bifocals are simply an alternative to wearing separate glasses for distance and reading. This includes a progressive, or "no line," bifocal. Another variation is a trifocal, which provides intermediate near vision as well. People who see well in the distance without glasses sometimes still prefer bifocals so that they don't have to take their reading glasses on and off.

IS THERE ANY WAY TO TELL ME EXACTLY WHAT MY VISION WILL BE WITHOUT GLASSES AFTER CATARACT SURGERY?

Unfortunately, because of the cataract's presence, it is impossible to demonstrate this to you. This makes it particularly difficult to decide on certain options, such as a multifocal IOL. Furthermore, the decision usually hinges on the targeted focal distance. Remember that your surgeon cannot precisely control or necessarily achieve the exact focal distance targeted.

What Is a Secondary Membrane?

A small percentage of people (less than 20%) who undergo cataract surgery may develop what is called a *secondary membrane*, posterior capsular opacification, or "secondary cataract." However, the term *secondary cataract* is a misnomer because cataracts do not grow back. Recall that the lens implant is supported by the original lens capsule, so that the patient is looking through both the IOL and the transparent back part of the lens capsule. A secondary membrane consists of a thin layer of cloudy cells that accumulates on and gradually covers the back of the lens capsule much like dust collecting on a window (Figure CA-8). As a result, light cannot be focused clearly through this cloudy capsule, and the individual has a gradual, progressive decline in vision. The most common symptoms are blurred or hazy vision; one may also experience glare. Patients with a significant membrane usually say that their vision is not as good as it was right after they recovered from their cataract surgery. A secondary membrane typically occurs 1 to 3 years after cataract surgery. Such a membrane is more likely to occur in younger patients and those who have had subcapsular cataracts, the ones that form along the back of the human lens. Fortunately, this condition is not a complication and is not serious.

Treating a Secondary Membrane

If you develop a secondary membrane, it is easily treated. A painless procedure known as a *YAG capsulotomy* is performed in a matter of minutes in a surgery center or an office. YAG is short for Nd:YAG and refers to neodymium:yttrium-aluminum-garnet crystals that are the active medium in the laser used. This procedure may be advisable if a hazy capsule has caused a progressive, bothersome blur.

For a YAG laser treatment, you will be seated at an eye microscope similar to that used for a routine eye examination. Anesthetic drops are all that will be needed to numb your eye.

A special focusing lens may be placed on your eye to control eye movements and to prevent the lids from closing. Because the amount of laser energy is so small, there is no danger to your other eye or other parts of your body. Although you should not feel any pain, you will notice a clicking sound as the laser is administered (Figure CA-9). This series of multiple clicks represents the many tiny applications used to create a small opening in the cloudy capsule (Figure CA-10). Each microscopic nick will result in a progressively larger opening until the optimal size is attained.

Following the treatment, your eye may be temporarily blurred for a few hours. You may also notice new temporary floaters. Your eye may be slightly irritated later in the day. Pain is uncommon, and a bandage is not necessary. You may notice improvement in your vision later on that same day or by the next morning. The laser treatment does not change your eyeglass prescription.

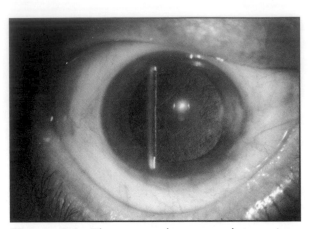

Figure 7-1. The secondary membrane is a clouding of the back lens capsule behind the artificial lens and has a ground glass appearance in this photo. The clear opening in the middle was made with the YAG laser.

The procedure will never have to be repeated because the optical hole in the capsule will always remain open (Figure 7-1).

DOES A YAG PROCEDURE CARRY RISKS?

Fortunately, risks for this procedure are minimal. In fact, the laser procedure avoids risks associated with incisional surgery, such as bleeding or infection. Rarely, in predisposed eyes, changes in the eye fluid pressure and in the retina can occur after the laser procedure. You may notice floaters immediately following the laser treatment. These are microscopic particles from the capsule and will disappear. They are different from the permanent floaters in the vitreous gel that most patients develop as a result of aging.

Chapter 8

Reducing Dependence on Eyeglasses

Having cataract surgery should certainly improve your vision, and it can reduce your need for eyeglasses. However, you will still need glasses at times. Here's why: When we are young, the focusing muscles inside our eye change and control the shape of our natural lens. This natural focusing ability is called *accommodation* and enables our eye to shift its focus from far to near, like an auto-focus camera.

Unfortunately, the eye's natural lens hardens as we age. As it loses flexibility, we gradually lose our accommodation. *Presbyopia* is the name for the normal loss of this far-to-near focusing ability due to age. By our mid 40s, we must start to use reading glasses, bifocals, or trifocals.

Chang DF, Lee BS.
*Cataracts: A Patient's Guide to Treatment,
Third Edition* (pp 81-91).
© 2016 SLACK Incorporated.

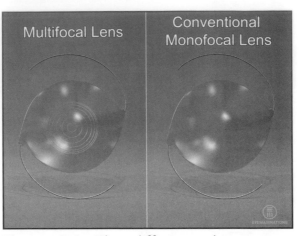

Figure 8-1. The difference between a multifocal and a monofocal lens.

The conventional monofocal intraocular lens (IOL) is a single-focus lens that optimizes focus at one distance. For most patients, this lens will likely provide good distance vision without glasses; however, it cannot provide far-distance focus one moment and near focus the next. Various refractive IOLs, first described in Chapter 4, are popular options that can reduce your dependence on eyeglasses compared to a conventional monofocal IOL but require additional costs that are not covered by health insurance (Figure 8-1).

Presbyopia:
How Multifocal IOLs May Help

The multifocal IOLs are sometimes referred to as *presbyopia-correcting* IOLs and will reduce the need to wear reading glasses compared to a monofocal IOL. With multifocal IOLs, part of the lens is set for distance focus and part of the lens is set for near focus. This means that there will likely be reasonably good near and far vision without glasses.

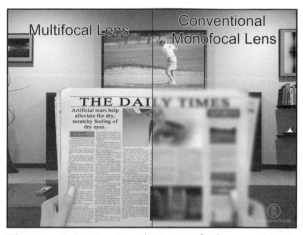

Figure 8-2. A simulation of the patient's view through a multifocal IOL (left) and a monofocal IOL (right).

The design is entirely different from bifocal eyeglasses, in which the top portion is designed for distance and the bottom area for near. With a multifocal IOL, the brain automatically finds the correct focus. Having to take their reading glasses on and off frequently to read something momentarily is inconvenient for many people. Although the multifocal IOL will not totally eliminate the need for reading glasses, it should give patients the convenience of reading many things at near—such as a wristwatch, price tags, cookbooks, magazines, mail, and menus—without the inconvenience of having to put on reading glasses (Figure 8-2).

It's important to note, however, that not everyone with a multifocal lens implant can read equally well without glasses and that it is impossible to know in advance how often a person will need to wear glasses after receiving a multifocal IOL. This technology generally works best when a patient has a multifocal IOL in each eye but still provides convenience when the patient only needs cataract surgery in one eye. Further, there are some trade-offs to consider with a multifocal IOL. The different focal zones of the lens create the appearance of thin rings or halos around lights at night, when the pupils naturally become larger. These halos are much less problematic than those caused by cataracts and are less noticeable with the newer multifocal IOL designs.

The halos do not obscure the vision. They become less noticeable and distracting over time; the brain learns to ignore them the same way it learns to ignore background noise, such as traffic sounds or an air-conditioning fan. So when are multifocal lenses not recommended?

These IOLs do not work well if there is too much astigmatism or other problems involving the cornea, retina, or optic nerve. Aside from these issues, your lifestyle and activities should be considered, along with the additional cost. Reducing the need to wear glasses is not a priority for everyone, and the multifocal IOL might not be as appealing for these individuals.

Presbyopia: How Pseudoaccommodating IOLs May Help

Pseudoaccommodating IOLs are another type of presbyopia-correcting lens. Compared to a monofocal or "single-focus" lens, these IOLs are designed to provide a wider range or depth of focus without glasses. This greater focusing range is created by the optics of the IOL rather than by having the artificial lens change shape like a young human lens. Recall that the latter natural focusing mechanism is called *accommodation*, so these IOLs are called *pseudoaccommodating*—they reduce dependence on eyeglasses by simulating some degree of natural focusing ability. However, this benefit may vary among

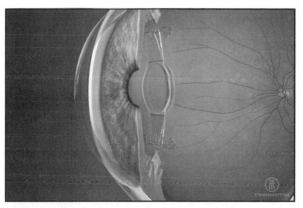

Figure 8-3. A pseudoaccommodating IOL is designed to increase the range of focus compared to a conventional IOL.

individual eyes, and one should not expect them to eliminate the need for glasses entirely (Figure 8-3).

Like the pre-presbyopic natural lens, pseudoaccommodating IOLs generally increase one's focus for midrange distances such as the car dashboard or a desktop computer. They are less likely to provide near (reading) focus than multifocal IOLs, which have a different optical design.

As with multifocal IOLs, the additional costs are not covered by insurance, and too much astigmatism will decrease the effectiveness of this IOL. Most individuals with pseudoaccommodating IOLs will still need to wear eyeglasses for seeing at certain distances. One way to improve the ability to see without glasses with pseudoaccommodating IOLs is to have one eye focused better for far distance and the other eye focused slightly closer for near.

LASIK as an Enhancement Procedure

For both the multifocal or pseudoaccommodating IOLs to work well, it is particularly important for the selected lens power to match the optics of the eye. Despite flawless surgery, some patients are still unable to see as well as they would like without glasses. If this is due to the lens power being "off," what can be done? Aside from wearing glasses or contact lenses, a theoretical solution might be to exchange the refractive IOL for another lens with a different power. However, because of the difficulty and risks associated with removing an IOL, it is usually safer to perform an enhancement using the external laser procedure known as *LASIK*. In a LASIK procedure, the curvature of the cornea is reshaped with a computerized laser beam. Note that a LASIK enhancement is a separate, elective procedure that should be delayed for several months after cataract surgery. The chance of needing this enhancement after receiving either multifocal or pseudoaccommodating IOLs is not high, but it is greater in patients with higher astigmatism or in those who have previously needed strong prescription eyeglasses.

Astigmatism:
How Astigmatic Keratotomy May Help

Astigmatic keratotomy is another procedure that may be used to reduce the need for eyeglasses. As you may recall reading in an earlier chapter, astigmatism is a common refractive error that results from an inborn imperfect optical shape of the cornea, the clear front window of the eye. In astigmatism, the shape of the cornea is oblong rather than round (Figure 8-4). As a result, the cornea will misfocus details and cause blurry vision that is corrected by wearing eyeglasses. The more astigmatism

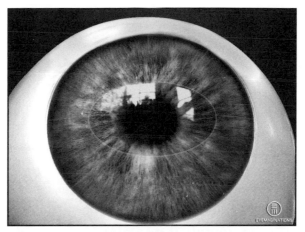

Figure 8-4. Astigmatism is an optical blur caused by the shape of the cornea being more oval than round.

you have, the more blurry your vision will be without eyeglasses.

Astigmatism can be reduced with astigmatic keratotomy. To perform this procedure, a surgeon uses special surgical blades to make tiny slits in the surface of the oblong cornea, allowing the cornea to become more rounded in shape and improving the natural focus. By varying the length, depth, and location of the incisions, an ophthalmologist can control how much change is made in the cornea's shape and curvature.

Astigmatic keratotomy is a separate procedure from cataract removal. However, because the small incisions for astigmatic keratotomy are made in the cornea's external surface, this procedure can be done safely at the same time as cataract surgery. It's fairly common to have both procedures done at the same time, as this does not prolong the postoperative recovery time and does not increase the overall risk of cataract surgery. Your surgeon will generally advise you of any specific risks for undergoing astigmatic keratotomy based on your particular situation.

Although astigmatic keratotomy usually will not eliminate astigmatism completely, it can help you see more clearly without eyeglasses. Even if glasses are needed, the patient will likely not need as strong of a lens prescription. Interestingly, this procedure is more effective the older you are. Why? The stiffness in the cornea increases with age, which increases the effectiveness of the tiny slits made in the surface of the cornea.

Astigmatic keratotomy is a safe procedure and is worth considering if your ophthalmologist thinks you are a candidate and you are interested in enhancing your ability to see without glasses. Note that, as an elective refractive procedure, the cost of astigmatic keratotomy is not covered by health insurance.

Astigmatism:
How Toric IOLs May Help

A special type of monofocal lens known as a *toric IOL* is designed to improve astigmatism. The toric lens incorporates the optical astigmatism correction that would otherwise need to be worn in eyeglasses or contact lenses directly into the IOL. Like the eyeglass prescription for astigmatism, it is aligned according to the location of astigmatism on the cornea (Figure 8-5).

To correct blurred vision, the toric IOL accomplishes 2 things. First, the *amount* of astigmatism-correcting power of the IOL is matched to the amount of astigmatism of the cornea. Second, the *orientation* of the astigmatism correction of the IOL is aligned with the cornea's astigmatism. As a result, the natural eyesight without

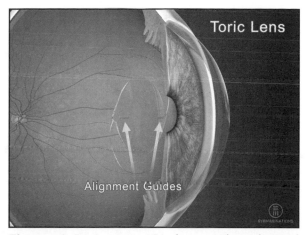

Figure 8-5. A toric IOL has to be aligned in order to correct and neutralize the eye's astigmatism.

glasses is improved with a toric IOL. The toric IOL may not correct all of the astigmatism, especially if it is severe; eyeglasses or contact lenses can correct whatever astigmatism remains.

In addition, because the toric IOL is a monofocal lens, reading glasses must still be worn if the decision is made to aim for good distance eyesight. Toric IOLs cost more than conventional IOLs, and the additional cost is not covered by insurance.

Which IOL Is Right for You?

It can be confusing to have so many different types of IOLs to choose from. Your options in this arena—such as whether a multifocal or pseudoaccommodating IOL is right for you or whether you should have astigmatism reduction—is something that you and your eye doctor should decide together. Whether or not you should take

Whether or not you should take extra steps to reduce your need for eyeglasses is a personal decision. extra steps to reduce your need for eyeglasses is a personal decision. Start by evaluating how strong your desire is to reduce your need for glasses.

Based on your eye examination and your goals, your ophthalmologist will be able to recommend the best type of IOL for you. Remember that multifocal, pseudoaccommodating, toric, and conventional monofocal IOLs will all provide excellent vision following cataract surgery. The difference is in what you can see when you aren't wearing glasses.

Intraoperative Aberrometry

As discussed in Chapter 4, the surgeon takes multiple preoperative measurements to choose the IOL power that is most likely to deliver the intended result. An intraoperative technology called *aberrometry* allows the doctor to make additional measurements during the surgery. This equipment is integrated into the operating microscope and can be used to help guide IOL selection. Intraoperative aberrometry may be particularly valuable in patients who are receiving a multifocal, pseudoaccommodating, or toric IOL or who have had prior refractive surgery such as LASIK or photorefractive keratectomy. Additionally, the same aberrometer can help with correction of astigmatism by providing immediate feedback on astigmatic keratotomies and placement of a toric IOL.

Femtosecond Laser Refractive Cataract Surgery

At the time of this writing, the femtosecond laser is being evaluated to see whether it can be used to enhance the refractive results of cataract surgery. This laser is able to cut tissue and can be used at the time of cataract surgery to perform astigmatic keratotomy.

Current studies have failed to show any generalized safety benefit from use of the femtosecond laser. Moreover, the additional cost is not covered by insurance. There is widespread agreement that this technology is not necessary for excellent results with cataract surgery. Depending on their surgical technique and level of experience, surgeons have varying opinions about the pros and cons of this technology for cataract surgery.

All figures in Chapter 8 have been reprinted with permission from Eyemaginations.

Chapter 9

Special Conditions and Cataract Surgery

I f you have health problems such as diabetes or other eye conditions such as glaucoma, high myopia, or macular degeneration, you may be concerned your condition will make you a poor candidate for cataract surgery. It is important to realize that if some of your vision loss is due to another eye condition, cataract surgery may not result in as much vision improvement as you were hoping for. On the other hand, advances in technology and the skill of your surgeon may still allow you to reap many of the benefits of cataract surgery. Each situation must be evaluated on an individual basis. Your doctor will

Your doctor will discuss the proper timing of surgery and how other eye or health conditions may influence the outcome of your cataract surgery.

Chang DF, Lee BS.
Cataracts: A Patient's Guide to Treatment,
Third Edition (pp 93-112).
© 2016 SLACK Incorporated.

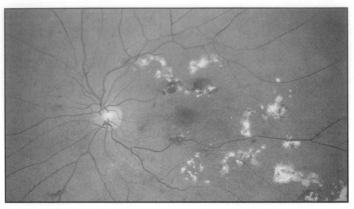

Figure 9-1. Diabetic retinopathy with leaking blood vessels.

discuss the proper timing of surgery and how other eye or health conditions may influence the outcome of your cataract surgery.

Diabetes

If you have diabetes, you already know that it is a medical condition that results in abnormally high levels of blood sugar. It is estimated that 29 million Americans, or 9% of the population, have diabetes. People with diabetes are 60% more likely to develop cataracts and tend to develop them at an earlier age than they otherwise might.

CHECKING FOR RETINOPATHY

If you have diabetes and you have a cataract, your ophthalmologist will conduct a careful preoperative evaluation of your eye. The doctor will be checking for a condition known as *diabetic retinopathy*, which refers to cumulative damage to small blood vessels in the retina caused by elevated blood sugar levels (Figure 9-1). Today, with proper medication and prompt eye treatment, most diabetics will not lose their vision to retinopathy.

If you have diabetes but do not have diabetic retinopathy, you should still expect an excellent outcome from cataract surgery. People with diabetes about to undergo operations elsewhere in the body are often told that they may not heal as well as people without diabetes. Fortunately, this is not the case with small-incision cataract surgery; the incision is so small that healing is rapid even for patients with diabetes.

DETERMINING THE SEVERITY OF RETINOPATHY

If you have diabetic retinopathy, the prognosis for cataract surgery depends on the severity of the condition. There are 2 forms of retinopathy: nonproliferative and proliferative. In the more common form, nonproliferative diabetic retinopathy, the capillaries in the retina become leaky and porous over time, potentially causing the leakage of small amounts of clear fluid called *edema* into the surrounding retina. If enough fluid seeps into the macula at the center of the retina, the central vision will become blurry. Macular edema is currently the most common retinal cause of impaired vision in people with diabetes. Drug or laser treatment directed toward the macula may be able to halt or slow this process.

Proliferative diabetic retinopathy is potentially even more serious. The damaged blood vessels start to narrow and eventually close off, resulting in poor circulation to the areas of retina that they feed. As a result, abnormal new blood vessels start to grow from the surface of the retina into the adjacent vitreous gel. These abnormal vessels can either bleed into the vitreous or form scars that lead to retinal detachments. If detected early enough, these proliferations of abnormal blood vessels can be halted by laser therapy.

For someone with active or worsening diabetic retinopathy, it is better to delay cataract surgery until after any necessary retinal treatment has been performed and the retinopathy is stabilized. It is also important to have one's blood sugar under control. When the retinopathy is advancing and unstable, especially if the blood sugar control is poor, cataract surgery can actually worsen the blood vessel complications and leakage.

PROCEEDING WITH CATARACT SURGERY

Once the retinopathy has been stabilized, can one proceed with cataract surgery? The surgery can remove the cataract, but it can't reverse vision impairment caused by the diabetic retinopathy. If this impairment is mild, cataract surgery can still provide reasonably good vision. However, if the retinal damage is extensive, the person's vision will still be quite limited, even after cataract surgery. Any retinal damage would also make a multifocal intraocular lens (IOL) unlikely to be successful.

In some cases, the eye doctor may want to remove the cataract because it interferes with the ability to diagnose and treat the diabetic retinopathy. Unfortunately, the surgeon can't know in advance just how much the pre-existing retinal disease impairs vision. If you have diabetic retinopathy and a cataract, talk with your ophthalmologist about whether surgery will provide a significant improvement in your vision.

Glaucoma

Because glaucoma and cataracts are very common in older people, it's not surprising that many people have

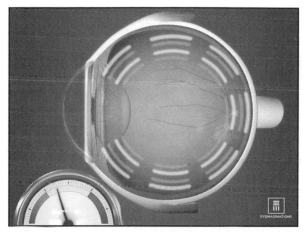

Figure 9-2. The eye is filled with circulating fluid that keeps the eyeball inflated under a reasonably constant fluid pressure.

both conditions. As discussed in Chapter 3, glaucoma is caused by excessive fluid pressure within the eyeball. How does this occur? A clear fluid, the aqueous humor, constantly circulates inside the front of the eyeball (Figure 9-2). This fluid normally drains through a tiny sieve-like drain at the base of the iris; however, over time this drain can clog, and because the fluid can no longer exit as quickly, an elevated pressure inside the eyeball results (Figure 9-3). The total amount of fluid is extremely small, only about one-sixteenth teaspoon, so there are no noticeable symptoms, and you absolutely can't feel the elevated pressure.

If the fluid pressure is not lowered, it can cause gradual and permanent damage to the optic nerve (Figure 9-4). Glaucoma is often treated with eye drop medications or a laser procedure to reduce the eye pressure to a safe level. Sometimes more extensive surgery is required.

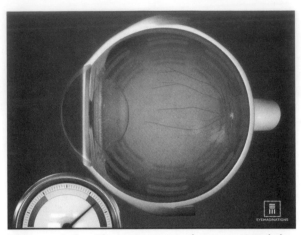

Figure 9-3. Glaucoma is characterized by elevated fluid pressure within the eye.

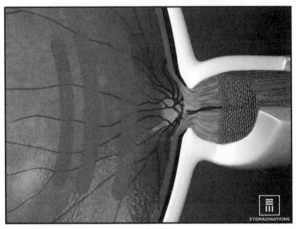

Figure 9-4. Prolonged elevation of eye fluid pressure over time can gradually and permanently damage the optic nerve.

CAN YOU HAVE CATARACT SURGERY?

One of the questions that virtually every glaucoma patient asks is, "Does having glaucoma lower my chances for successful cataract surgery?" Most glaucoma patients who do not have significant vision loss can expect good results from cataract surgery. It is important to realize that any vision loss due to advanced glaucoma is permanent, and that portion of the vision impairment cannot be restored with cataract surgery.

Most people should continue their glaucoma drops immediately before and after cataract surgery. Occasionally, some may be asked to temporarily stop or change a particular glaucoma medication. Patients often are concerned that cataract surgery will aggravate their glaucoma. Cataract surgery patients with glaucoma may experience variable eye pressure for a while following cataract surgery, but this is normal and only temporary. Generally, cataract surgery does nothing to worsen glaucoma. In fact, the eye pressure frequently decreases after small-incision cataract surgery.

COMBINING SURGERY FOR CATARACTS AND GLAUCOMA

Most people with glaucoma will never need traditional glaucoma surgery. However, it is possible that your doctor will determine that, in addition to cataract surgery, you may also need a surgical procedure such as a trabeculectomy to keep your glaucoma from progressing. This surgery is performed to decrease the risk of damage to the optic nerve by lowering eye pressure, and it can be done at the same time as cataract surgery.

In a trabeculectomy, the surgeon makes a tiny, permanent, valve-like drain in the eye wall to bypass the clogged natural drainage area. You may wonder what keeps such an incision from scarring and healing shut. To keep the valve open, drugs are applied at the time of surgery that essentially prevent the valve from being scarred shut.

Although a trabeculectomy can improve the long-term control of glaucoma, combining the procedures may delay visual recovery from the cataract surgery. Vision may remain blurred for several months or more, especially if the eye pressure is initially very low. In addition, there are some risks associated with trabeculectomy, such as lowering the eye pressure too much.

Recently, microscopic drainage devices have been developed for glaucoma patients. These tiny permanently implanted tubes, called *stents*, are designed to lower eye pressure by increasing the rate of fluid outflow through the eyeball's natural drainage area. They can be inserted during cataract surgery, do not carry the same risks associated with a trabeculectomy, and should not affect the vision or the recovery of the eye. By improving eye pressure control, these microscopic drainage stents may reduce the number of medications that a person with glaucoma must take.

High Myopia

As explained in an earlier chapter, myopia refers to being nearsighted—you can see things up close without glasses, but you need glasses or contact lenses to see clearly in the distance. Those who become severely nearsighted at an early age are called *high myopes*. The length of the eye is measured from the front, at the cornea, to the back, where the retina is located. Like feet, eyeballs come in different lengths, and those with high myopia have longer eyeballs that are shaped more like an egg than a ping-pong ball.

There are several special considerations for cataracts in high myopes. First, cataracts in young myopic patients may be more difficult to diagnose in their earliest stage. Second, these individuals are at a slightly increased risk for retinal detachment occurring during their lifetime.

DIAGNOSING EARLY CATARACTS IN HIGH MYOPES

Individuals with long myopic eyes have a tendency to form cataracts at an earlier age, sometimes even in their 40s or 50s. These early myopic cataracts are called *oil droplet cataracts* because they resemble a tiny oil droplet in the center of the lens of the eye. One of the common symptoms of this type of cataract is double vision, or seeing ghost images from light sources at night. An example would be seeing multiple moons in the night sky. As these cataracts progress, they change the optics of the eye such that the myopia increases quite rapidly.

The early symptoms of these cataracts may be quite subtle, and their presence may not be entirely obvious during an eye examination. Younger patients are not expected to have cataracts, nor do these cataracts resemble those found in older patients. As a result, these early oil droplet cataracts may escape diagnosis initially.

At first, stronger eyeglass prescriptions can compensate for the increased myopia caused by the cataract. However, as the cataracts get progressively worse, the myopia increases more rapidly. Vision, even with new glasses, remains poor.

RETINAL DETACHMENT IN HIGH MYOPES

Over the course of their lifetime, individuals with highly myopic eyes are more susceptible to retinal detachment, the sudden separation of the retina from the inner wall of the eyeball (Figure 9-5). Why? In the longer

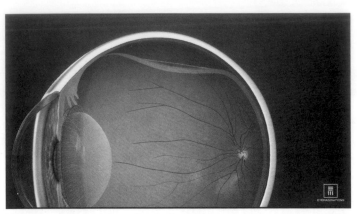

Figure 9-5. In a retinal detachment, the thin retina separates from the inner wall of the eye. This must be surgically repaired to avoid blindness.

myopic eye, the sclera and retina are more stretched, which may cause microscopic weak spots in the peripheral retina that are predisposed to tearing. The precipitating factor is the natural aging of the vitreous humor, a transparent, gel-like substance that occupies the central cavity within our eyeballs and becomes more watery with age. Much like gelatin that has started to liquefy, the vitreous humor tends to slosh around with eye movement the more watery it becomes.

Although retinal detachments are more likely to occur in highly myopic people than in the rest of the population, the actual odds of this occurring are still very small, less than 5%. However, the risk of retinal detachment in predisposed eyes increases slightly during the years following even uncomplicated cataract surgery. This is particularly true of young myopic men. The mechanism most likely relates to the fact that the artificial lens is much thinner than the natural lens. Cataract surgery therefore creates additional space for the aging vitreous humor to slosh about.

Fortunately, if the cataract is significant, the benefits of surgery still outweigh the risks. People with severe myopia garner one additional major benefit from cataract surgery because the IOL powers selected for them can dramatically improve their ability to see without glasses. When they need cataract surgery in the second eye, some of these patients are actually pleased because they are looking forward to this improvement in their severely nearsighted refraction. Although highly myopic patients will likely still need glasses for many tasks, they will have good functional vision for many everyday tasks without glasses for the first time in their adult lives.

IOL SELECTION IN HIGH MYOPES (AND HYPEROPES)

As discussed in Chapter 4, your surgeon will take multiple measurements of your eyes before performing your cataract surgery. Those measurements are then incorporated into various formulas to calculate the IOL power that is used inside your eye. Fortunately, improvements in both the measurement technology and the formulas that are used have improved the accuracy of IOL selection.

However, the formulas are more precise for patients whose eye dimensions are in the typical range. You may remember from the earlier discussion that the formulas are estimating where the IOL will sit inside the eye and therefore the amount of focusing power it will provide after surgery. The estimate is more difficult in those eyes with high myopia (nearsightedness) or hyperopia (farsightedness).

Macular Degeneration

The macula is the small central area of the retina where fine vision and detail are captured (Figure 9-6). Like other parts of our body, it can become weaker with age. It

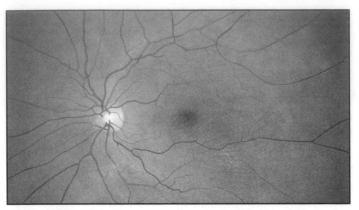

Figure 9-6. This is a normal macula. The macula is the darker area in the center. The round, white structure located to the left is the optic nerve, where it attaches into the back of the eyeball. The major blood vessels of the retina enter and exit through the optic nerve but do not run directly through the macula.

is estimated that 15 million Americans have some degree of macular degeneration. This is a general term that covers the entire spectrum of aging change to the macula. Most people will only have milder degrees of macular degeneration and will not experience major vision loss. Even people with the most severe form of macular degeneration never go completely blind. Although they may lose central vision, they maintain good peripheral vision. Much like age-related hearing loss, vision changes from macular degeneration usually occur very gradually.

Some people with macular degeneration may experience a more rapid decline of their central vision because of a complication called *neovascularization*. This refers to the growth of abnormal blood vessels underneath the weakened macula that eventually start to leak fluid or blood. These abnormal leaking blood vessels can be treated with an injection of medication, but they may

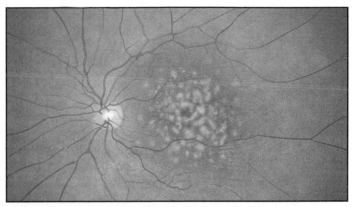

Figure 9-7. This is dry macular degeneration. The whitish spots are called *drusen,* and this appearance indicates significant aging changes within the macula.

permanently damage and scar the macular retinal cells. If these abnormal leaking blood vessels are discovered, the patient is said to have wet macular degeneration. As long as these abnormal vessels have not formed, the patient is said to have dry macular degeneration (Figure 9-7).

CAN YOU HAVE CATARACT SURGERY IF YOU HAVE MACULAR DEGENERATION?

Whether macular degeneration affects one's chances for successful cataract surgery is a matter of some confusion. If the cataract is advanced enough, macular degeneration patients can certainly benefit from having it removed. The surgery should not affect the macular degeneration—the macula is at the back of the eye, and the cataract is closer to the front of the eye. However, how well one sees following cataract surgery depends on the portion of vision loss caused by the macular degeneration. For example, if you have mild macular degeneration and an advanced cataract, you should still experience a significant improvement in your vision after surgery. On the other hand, if you have advanced macular degeneration and a mild cataract, you may not see much improvement in your vision at all.

Your doctor will try to determine whether the cataract is significant enough to warrant surgery, although it's impossible to know in advance to what degree your symptoms are caused by the cataract vs the macular degeneration; it isn't possible before surgery to test separately the vision loss from the 2 coexisting conditions. Many people who have both conditions undergo cataract surgery to get whatever partial vision improvement they can. Only then will they have the satisfaction of knowing that they've done everything possible to maximize their vision.

The more serious, wet form of macular degeneration can develop at any time, including in patients who have undergone cataract surgery. However, more recent evidence shows that cataract surgery does not appear to increase the risk of developing wet macular degeneration.

Previous Refractive Surgery

In the previous chapter, we discussed a form of refractive surgery known as *LASIK*, which improves distance vision by reshaping the cornea with a laser. In the early 1980s, prior to LASIK, another refractive surgery procedure, radial keratotomy, was the primary method used to treat nearsightedness. Unlike LASIK, radial keratotomy involved making multiple spoke-like incisions in the cornea to reshape it. Nowadays, radial keratotomy has been almost completely replaced by LASIK surgery, which achieves better and more stable results. (The radial keratotomy procedure should not be confused with astigmatic keratotomy, which is an excellent method to treat astigmatism.)

If you have had either of these forms of refractive surgery in the past (including photorefractive keratotomy, or PRK, a surgery similar to LASIK), you might wonder how the procedure may affect your having cataract surgery. You can still have cataract surgery using the same state-of-the-art techniques and IOLs; however, your doctor must be prepared to deal with a special problem created by the refractive surgery. Because refractive procedures reshape the cornea, it becomes difficult to measure the power of the cornea properly before cataract surgery. The resulting inaccurate measurements make it much harder for the doctor to calculate the appropriate power for the IOL.

If you've had refractive surgery, your ophthalmologist will make the best estimate of the optimum IOL power using a combination of supplemental techniques. It is very beneficial to have your medical records containing the pre- and postoperative data from your previous refractive surgery. As mentioned in Chapter 4, a technology called *intraoperative aberrometry* can take additional measurements of your eye during the cataract surgery. This may be very helpful for choosing the IOL power in patients with prior refractive surgery.

The further off the calculations are, the stronger your postoperative distance vision glasses will need to be. It's uncommon, but if the IOL power calculation is too far off, it may be necessary to exchange the IOL implant or perhaps to "piggyback" an additional IOL on top of the first one.

It is recommended that you provide your cataract surgeon with your medical records that provide information about your vision both before and after any previous refractive surgeries.

Complicated Eyes

A complicated eye refers to one that presents a variety of difficulties for cataract surgery. It may have certain anatomic features, such as small pupils, that complicate the steps of the surgery. Or the cataract may have characteristics that make it more challenging to remove, such as mature brown and white cataracts. Although a number of factors can make cataract surgery more difficult in some eyes, when you are in experienced hands, the prognosis is still generally excellent.

SMALL PUPILS

For a variety of reasons, a number of patients have pupils that do not dilate very widely after the dilating drops are given. Cataract surgeons refer to these patients as having small pupils. In some individuals the pupil size becomes smaller with age or after taking glaucoma drops such as pilocarpine. Other patients have small pupils as a result of taking drugs such as Flomax (tamsulosin) for prostate enlargement. This family of drugs, called *alpha blockers*, ends with the suffix *-osin* (eg, silodosin, doxazosin, terazosin, prazosin, or alfuzosin) and can lead to *floppy iris syndrome*, which can cause cataract surgery to be more difficult. It is important to inform your doctor if you are taking or have ever taken any drugs for prostate conditions.

Smaller pupils make intraocular surgery more challenging by providing less working room for the surgeon inside the eye. This increases the chance of tearing the capsular bag, which may require the use of an alternate style of IOL. Fortunately, a surgeon is able to expand or widen the pupil temporarily, making it easier to remove the cataract and allowing most patients with small pupils to have a good outcome. Patients with small pupils or floppy iris syndrome should know that there is a small risk of injury to the iris or change in the pupil shape.

WEAK CAPSULAR BAG AND ZONULES

Modern cataract surgery involves preserving the transparent capsular bag that surrounds the eye's lens so that it will permanently support the IOL. Microscopic support ligaments known as *zonules* securely suspend the lens and its capsular bag behind the iris. However, weak or deficient zonules can complicate cataract removal. In addition, the capsular bag itself may be too weak to support the artificial lens implant.

A number of factors increase the risk of having weak zonules or a weak capsular bag. Eye injuries or prior eye surgery, such as glaucoma or retina surgery, can stretch or weaken the support ligaments. People who have an eye condition called *retinopathy of prematurity*, a result of premature birth, often have weak support ligaments. Advanced age may also cause the support ligaments to become fragile.

Another common cause of weak or deficient support ligaments, especially among older Whites, is called *pseudoexfoliation.* Particularly common among people of Northern European, Russian, or Scandinavian descent, this aging condition causes microscopic white deposits on the eye's iris and lens that can be seen only with the slit lamp examination. With pseudoexfoliation, the capsular bag can be more fragile and more prone to developing tears during surgery. Many people with this condition also have smaller pupils and a higher risk of developing glaucoma.

In many cases, the surgeon has no way of knowing about a weak capsular bag or weak support ligaments before surgery, although a few subtle clinical signs may arouse suspicion. During surgery, the surgeon can tell whether a weakness exists by how the lens behaves during the surgical steps. Once aware of the condition, he or she can use alternative techniques to place the IOL in the eye and still achieve good results. If the zonules are very weak, a microscopic plastic ring can be permanently inserted into the capsular bag to stabilize it.

MATURE BROWN CATARACTS

When certain types of cataracts become very advanced, they become hard and solid, and the central core starts to turn brown or even black. A mature brown cataract is more difficult to remove because it takes more ultrasound energy to break it into small pieces for removal. Both the density of the lens and the use of greater ultrasound energy may increase the stresses applied to the zonules and the capsular bag during surgery. This can increase the risk of a tear in the capsular bag. However, as discussed earlier, such a complication is manageable. On rare occasions, the surgeon may decide the cataract's core is too dense to be removed with phacoemulsification and choose to remove the cataract through a large-incision procedure.

Cataract surgery in these advanced cases should still yield a good outcome, but dense cataracts may make it difficult for the ophthalmologist to see the back of the eye to ensure that it is healthy before surgery. Because the surgery may take longer, the recovery of vision may be delayed by a few weeks.

MATURE WHITE CATARACTS

With some advanced cataracts, the entire lens turns white. This is the only time that cataracts change the

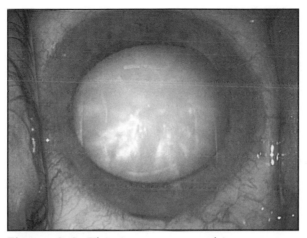

Figure 9-8. This is a mature white cataract. The eye cannot see anything because the entire lens has turned white.

external appearance of the eye. With these cataracts, the normally black pupil also appears white (Figure 9-8).

Mature white cataracts are more challenging to remove because they make it difficult for the surgeon to see the internal parts of the lens during surgery. The surgeon can use a special dye during the operation to help visualize the necessary lens structures. This type of cataract also carries a slightly higher risk for tearing the capsular bag. In addition, white cataracts make it impossible for the ophthalmologist to examine the back of the eyeball to see if other conditions, such as macular degeneration, might exist. If there are no other abnormalities with the retina or optic nerve, these patients should still achieve a good outcome from cataract surgery.

PEDIATRIC CATARACTS

We usually think of cataracts as a condition affecting the elderly. Most parents are surprised and puzzled if told that their infants or children have a cataract. Due to genetic or prenatal influences, babies may be born with a cataract affecting one or both eyes, and the density, size, and location can vary considerably. These factors determine whether and how urgently surgery is needed. Preoperative assessment may involve the child's pediatrician or a geneticist to check for associated diseases that may not have been previously diagnosed.

Pediatric ophthalmologists are specialists in diagnosing and treating eye diseases in children. Treating cataracts in children is much more complex than treating adults because the eye tissue changes as it matures. The fact that the immature eye will be changing in size so much in the first few years of life can make the use of IOLs in infants problematic. Parents should discuss with the surgeon the benefits of IOL placement in their child.

If cataract surgery is performed, postoperative care may include contact lens fitting, frequent modifications in the strength of glasses or contact lenses as the eye grows, and eye patching to manage a lazy eye.

Figures 9-2 through 9-5 have been reprinted with permission from Eyemaginations.

Conclusion

L earning for the first time that you have a cataract, an eye problem that will eventually require surgery, can be a frightening experience. As with any common medical condition, you probably have already heard plenty of piecemeal information from varying sources. Unfortunately, many people worry and delay surgery unnecessarily because of misunderstandings. Our goal in writing this book has been to give you detailed information and to help you understand as much about cataracts and surgery as possible.

The term *medical miracle* is probably overused. However, it is no exaggeration to say that cataract surgery with an artificial lens implant is one of the greatest successes in all of medicine and surgery. As we age, we are repeatedly frustrated to learn that for most natural aging ailments, our only hope is to slow or delay their progression. Fortunately, that is not the case with cataracts. Through this amazing, microsurgical outpatient procedure, we can halt an aging problem that is ruining your eyesight and permanently reverse it!

Cataract surgery is no longer something to avoid or dread. Thanks to modern technology and surgical innovation, the operation and the recovery have become much faster, safer, and easier. The most advanced cataract techniques have eliminated sutures, anesthetic injections, eye bandages, and postoperative restrictions for most

113

Chang DF, Lee BS.
Cataracts: A Patient's Guide to Treatment,
Third Edition (pp 113-114).
© 2016 SLACK Incorporated.

patients. Although these more advanced methods require a much greater level of skill and expertise on the part of the surgeon, cataract patients are the clear winners.

Cataract surgery is now the most commonly performed operation in the industrialized world, and millions of North Americans enjoy the benefits of renewed sight every year. The success rate is now among the highest of any operation performed anywhere in the body. Best of all, some people are surprised to find that afterward they are seeing better than they can remember. This is why many of our patients think back upon their cataract surgery as a gift. As eye surgeons, we feel equally blessed. Helping people regain vision they have lost is one of the most gratifying experiences that a physician can have.

We hope that the information we have presented is both interesting and reassuring to you. Taking the time to read and learn more about cataracts is a wise investment in your health. Becoming as knowledgeable as possible, having confidence in your surgeon, and having a positive attitude about your condition can help to make your overall surgical experience much easier.

Glossary

anterior capsule: The front of the transparent lens capsular bag, through which an opening must be made surgically in order to remove a cataract and implant an intraocular lens (IOL).

anterior chamber intraocular lens: IOL designed for implantation in front of the iris.

astigmatic keratotomy: Partial-thickness incisions in the cornea to improve its shape and decrease astigmatism.

astigmatism: Nonspherical shape of the cornea that causes blurring of the vision at all distances.

capsular bag: The transparent membrane surrounding the entire lens of the eyeball.

cataract: Loss of transparency of the natural lens.

combined procedure: Two separate operations being performed during the same sitting. In the context of cataracts, this usually refers to glaucoma or cornea surgery being performed coincidently with cataract surgery.

complicated eye: In the context of cataract surgery, this term refers to an eye that has anatomical features that make surgery more difficult.

conjunctiva: Thin, transparent mucous membrane that overlies the white sclera and lines the inner aspect of the upper and lower lids.

conjunctivitis: Inflammation of the conjunctiva. While this is a general term, it is often used in reference to an external eye infection.

Chang DF, Lee BS.
*Cataracts: A Patient's Guide to Treatment,
Third Edition* (pp 115-122).
© 2016 SLACK Incorporated.

cornea: Transparent, dome-shaped structure at the front of the eyeball through which all light rays enter the eye interior.

corneal clouding: Vision-impairing loss of corneal transparency. Depending upon the underlying cause and severity, this condition may be temporary or permanent.

cortical cataract: Type of cataract in which the haze is predominantly in the regions closest to the front and rear of the lens with a shape like spokes in a bicycle wheel.

diabetic retinopathy: Progressive retinal disorder that results from diabetes and the associated circulatory abnormalities.

diffuse cataract: A cataract in which the entire lens is uniformly hazy.

dilating drops: Medications administered as eye drops in order to expand the pupil temporarily. Used to permit visualization of the interior eye for either examination or surgery.

diopter: Standard optical unit of measure. In the context of eyes, this is the unit for measuring refractive error (nearsightedness, farsightedness, and astigmatism) or the power of prescription eyeglasses.

dry eye: Clinical term describing a relative lack of surface tear lubrication that typically results in symptoms of minor discomfort or fluctuating vision.

dry macular degeneration: See **macular degeneration**.

exfoliation (psuedoexfoliation): Asymptomatic eye condition characterized by microscopic changes visible during a dilated eye examination. Often associated with increased difficulty in performing cataract surgery due either to poor pupil dilation or weakness of the capsular bag support.

extracapsular surgery: Type of cataract surgery in which the capsular bag supporting the original lens is preserved in order to hold the IOL.

floater: Moving shadow in the field of vision. The usual cause is age-related liquefaction and clumping of the vitreous gel within the central ocular cavity.

floppy iris syndrome: Condition in which the iris billows during cataract surgery, also associated with a small pupil. Patients who take a class of medication called an *alpha blocker* are more likely to have this condition. Medications in this class include Flomax (tamsulosin) and other drugs for an enlarged prostate.

focal cataract: A cataract in which only portions of the lens are hazy.

foldable intraocular lens: IOL made of silicone or acrylic plastic to allow it to be folded for insertion through a small cataract incision.

free radicals: Chemical molecules implicated in damage to tissue. They may be caused by ultraviolet light.

general anesthesia: Type of anesthesia in which the patient is unconscious and a breathing tube connected to a respirator is used.

glaucoma: Eye disease characterized by progressive damage to the optic nerve. The usual cause is prolonged, abnormal elevation of the intraocular fluid pressure, which is treatable with medication or surgery.

halo: Symptom of rings appearing around point sources of light that is typically noticeable at night.

haptic: Flexible, wire-like support member of the IOL. The 2 haptics center the lens implant within the capsular support bag.

high myopia: Higher-than-average degree of nearsightedness associated with an elongated eyeball.

hyperopia: Refractive error in which light rays are mis-focused behind, rather than on, the retina. Called *farsightedness* because closer objects appear more blurred than distant objects, but patients with significant hyperopia have blurred vision at far as well.

intracapsular surgery: Cataract surgery in which the capsular bag is removed together with the lens. This is an older surgical technique that is not currently used.

intraocular lens (IOL): Artificial lens permanently implanted in the eye.

intraocular pressure: Internal fluid pressure of the eyeball. Prolonged elevation can lead to glaucoma.

intraoperative aberrometry: Technology that allows real-time measurement of the eye during surgery, providing guidance for IOL selection and positioning.

iris: The structure responsible for eye color that is located behind the cornea and functions like a curtain to regulate the amount of light that passes to the back of the eye.

LASIK (laser in situ keratomileusis): Refractive operation that involves laser-guided reshaping of the cornea beneath a thin, surgically created flap.

lens: Transparent intraocular tissue, located behind the pupil, that helps bring rays of light to a focus on the retina. When no longer transparent, this is called a *cataract.*

lidocaine: A common injectable anesthetic drug.

macula: Circular central-most region of the retina, which produces detailed, fine central vision.

macular degeneration: Age-related deterioration of the macula that impairs the central vision. If abnormal vessels grow and leak fluid beneath the weakened macula, the condition is called *wet.* If this has not occurred, the condition is called *dry.*

macular edema: Clear fluid collecting in the macula, which impairs central vision. The fluid source is abnormally porous capillaries in the retina.

mature brown cataract: Extremely advanced cataract stage in which the central nucleus becomes extremely solid.

mature white cataract: Extremely advanced cataract stage in which the lens turns white and becomes totally opaque.

monofocal intraocular lens: Type of IOL that provides optimal focus without glasses at a single distance.

monovision: Vision in which 2 eyes each see at different distances without glasses (have different refractive error). If achieved through contact lenses or IOLs, typically one eye sees better at a distance without glasses, and the second eye is focused closer without glasses.

multifocal intraocular lens: Type of IOL that provides optimal focus without glasses at more than one distance.

myopia: Refractive error in which light rays are misfocused in front of, rather than on, the retina. Called *nearsightedness* because without glasses, the patient sees clearer up close, but vision is blurry in the distance.

nonproliferative diabetic retinopathy: A form of retinopathy characterized by leaky, porous blood vessels.

nuclear cataract: Type of cataract in which the haze is predominantly in the center-most region of the lens.

oil droplet cataract: Type of nuclear cataract most often seen in young myopes, and so named because it looks like an oil droplet to the examining eye specialist.

ophthalmologist: A medical doctor (MD) who specializes in medical and surgical treatment of the eye. Ophthalmologists have graduated from medical school, a general medical or surgical internship, and ophthalmology residency. General ophthalmologists do not specialize and perform the majority of cataract surgeries. Specialist ophthalmologists receive extra training in the treatment of certain disorders such as those of the retina or cornea.

optic nerve: Nerve that transmits vision from the retina to the brain.

optician: Eye professional who is licensed to fit and dispense eyeglasses and sometimes contacts.

optometrist: Doctor of optometry (OD) specializing in vision problems, treating vision conditions with spectacles, contact lenses, and low vision aids and able to prescribe medications for certain eye diseases.

pediatric cataract: Cataract that develops in an infant or child.

phacoemulsification (phaco): Surgical technique in which the cataract is ultrasonically fragmented and aspirated.

pilocarpine: Glaucoma eye drop medication that also constricts the pupil.

pledget: Small thin sponge that can be placed just beneath the eyelid to administer eye medications.

posterior capsule: The back part of the transparent lens capsular bag, which is preserved in extracapsular cataract surgery in order to support the IOL.

posterior chamber intraocular lens: An IOL designed for implantation behind the iris.

presbyopia: Normal age-induced refractive error characterized by the inability to focus up close despite clear distance vision. Occurs after the age of 40 due to the normal loss of lens flexibility.

proliferative diabetic retinopathy: Form of retinopathy marked by abnormal, new blood vessels growing from the retina into the vitreous. These vessels can bleed or scar, leading to retinal detachment.

pseudoaccommodating intraocular lens: Type of IOL designed to provide partial focusing ability for improved range of vision without splitting the light into a distant and near image, as a multifocal IOL does.

pupil: Circular opening in the iris through which light passes in order to enter the back of the eye.

radial keratotomy: Refractive surgical procedure for myopia using radial cuts in the cornea.

refractive error: Optical imperfection in an otherwise healthy eye that results in blurred vision without glasses or contact lenses.

regional anesthesia: Type of local anesthesia in which anesthetic is injected around the eye.

retina: The thin, light-sensitive tissue that lines the back half of the eyeball and captures and registers vision.

retinal detachment: Condition in which the retina separates from the inner eye wall.

retinopathy of prematurity: Retinal condition associated with premature birth that carries a higher risk of retinal detachment.

sclera: The white wall of the eyeball.

secondary cataract: The clouding of the back of the posterior capsule months or years after cataract surgery. More accurately called a *secondary membrane* or *posterior capsular opacification*, the term is misleading because cataracts never recur.

secondary intraocular lens: An IOL that is inserted during a separate operation subsequent to the original cataract surgery.

secondary membrane: Condition in which the posterior capsule becomes cloudy months to years following successful cataract surgery.

small pupils: Eyes in which the pupil does not dilate normally following insertion of dilating drops.

Snellen chart: Standard eye chart for testing distance vision.

specialist ophthalmologist: See **ophthalmologist.**

speculum: Device that holds open the eyelids during eye surgery.

stye: Infected oil gland occurring in the edge of the eyelid.

toric intraocular lens: Type of IOL that has astigmatism correction built into it to compensate for imperfections in the corneal shape.

YAG capsulotomy: Laser procedure to create an opening in the posterior capsule when a secondary membrane is dense enough to affect vision.

Resources

American Council of the Blind
1703 N Beauregard Street, Suite 420
Alexandria, VA 22201
800-424-8666, 202 467-5081
www.acb.org

A membership organization that advocates for the blind and visually impaired. Offers information and referral service on all aspects of visual impairment and blindness. Website includes many resources for the visually impaired, including medical information on macular degeneration, catalogs, books, and related links.

American Foundation for the Blind
2 Penn Plaza, Suite 1102
New York, NY 10121
212-502-7600
www.afb.org

A national clearinghouse for information about blindness and visual impairment. Offers information for the visually impaired and publishes a Directory of Services for Blind and Visually Impaired Persons in the United States and Canada. Maintains regional offices. Website topics include aging and vision loss, education, employment, and technology. Also offers publications and links to other resources.

Chang DF, Lee BS.
Cataracts: A Patient's Guide to Treatment,
Third Edition (pp 123-130).
© 2016 SLACK Incorporated.

American Optometric Association
243 N Lindbergh Boulevard, Floor 1
St. Louis, MO 63141-7881
800-365-2219
www.aoa.org

Provides brochures on low vision and other eye problems. Website answers questions and offers consumer information, tips, and guidelines on eye exams, eye diseases, eye care, and eyewear.

Canadian National Institute for the Blind
800-563-2642
www.cnib.ca

Offers a wealth of information and tips for living with low vision, including a handbook for caregivers. Accessible in English or French.

The Center for the Partially Sighted
6101 W Centinela Avenue, Suite 150
Culver City, CA 90230
310-988-1970
www.low-vision.org

Counseling center offering support groups and counseling services for people who are vision impaired. Website offers information about warning signs and risk factors for vision loss.

Council of Citizens With Low Vision International
1703 N Beauregard Street, Suite 420
Alexandria, VA 22311-1746
800-773-2258
www.cclvi.org
Serves as an advocacy group for the visually impaired and provides information on low-vision technology. Publishes a newsletter.

EyeCare America
A Foundation of the American Academy of Ophthalmology
655 Beach Street
San Francisco, CA 94109
415-447-0381
www.aao.org/eyecare-america
Public service foundation of the American Academy of Ophthalmology. Free eye exams or glaucoma screenings offered to qualified individuals by member ophthalmologist volunteers. Free educational materials available on eye care. Order materials or request an eye exam by calling the helpline listed on the website.

EyeSmart
Developed by the American Academy of Ophthalmology
415-447-0213
www.aao.org/eye-health
Geared specifically toward patients, EyeSmart contains valuable information about eye diseases and conditions, featured articles related to eye health, and an interactive "Ask the Eye MD" question-and-answer forum. Eye health news, a featured video, and "Tip of the Day" are also provided.

Foundation Fighting Blindness
7168 Columbia Gateway Drive, Suite 100
Columbia, MD 21046
800-683-5555
www.blindness.org

An organization that funds research into retinal degenerative disease worldwide. Links to many other sites and organizations. Offers access to up-to-date information about eye diseases.

Glaucoma Research Foundation
251 Post Street, Suite 600
San Francisco, CA 94108
800-826-6693, 415-986-3162
www.glaucoma.org

The Glaucoma Research Foundation's mission is to preserve the sight and independence of individuals with glaucoma. The organization's main focus is public awareness about glaucoma and medical research to find a cure. The website provides information about glaucoma and how it is diagnosed and treated. A newsletter is also available.

Independent Living Services for Older Individuals Who Are Blind
www2.ed.gov/programs/rsailob/index.html

Federally funded program that offers free services to those aged 55 and older who have severe visual impairments. Recipients do not have to be totally blind to qualify. Program requirements vary from state to state. Log on to this website or contact your state's division of rehabilitation services for information.

Lighthouse Guild
15 W 65th Street
New York, NY 10023
800-284-4422
www.lighthouseguild.org

Provides information about vision impairment support groups, locating vision rehabilitation services nationwide, and free publications.

The Macula Foundation
210 E 64th Street
New York, NY 10065
800-622-8524, 212-605-3777
http://maculafoundation.org

A national support group that provides members with a newsletter and a phone hotline. Provides information and support for people with macular degeneration and other macular diseases.

Macular Degeneration Foundation
PO Box 531313
Henderson, NV 89053
888-633-3937, 702-450-2908 (Intl)
www.eyesight.org

Conducts research and educates patients on various aspects of retinal diseases. Website includes vision care specialists, books and tapes, research on nutrition, and links to other sites.

Macular Degeneration Partnership
17315 Studebaker Road, Suite 115
Cerritos, CA 90703
310-623-4466
www.amd.org

A coalition of patients, families, and leaders in the fields of vision and aging. Toll-free number has recorded information about age-related macular degeneration, 24 hours a day, 7 days a week. Website has information about macular degeneration, including the latest news on research and experimental treatments.

National Eye Institute, National Institutes of Health
National Eye Institute Information Office
31 Center Drive, MSC 2510
Bethesda, MD 20892-2510
301-496-5248
www.nei.nih.gov

Provides free information to the public about eye disease prevention, treatment, and research. Website features research results, disease information for patients, clinical studies, low-vision resources, and print and audio materials.

National Federation of the Blind
200 E Wells Street
Baltimore, MD 21230
410-659-9314
www.nfb.org

Provides referral and job services to the blind and visually impaired, as well as literature in a variety of formats. Website offers information about services, publications, and resources available to the blind and the vision impaired.

The Pediatric Glaucoma & Cataract Family Association
PO Box 144
27 St Clair Avenue E
Toronto, ON M4T 2L7
Canada
416-444-4536
www.pgcfa.org

Support organization for parents of children who have glaucoma or cataracts. The website provides information on pediatric glaucoma and cataracts via email, online forums, a free e-newsletter, and submitted questions to "Ask the Doc."

Prevent Blindness
211 W Wacker Drive, Suite 1700
Chicago, IL 60606
800-331-2020
www.preventblindness.org

Volunteer eye health and safety organization providing public and professional education, community programs, and research aimed at preventing blindness in America. Services include a toll-free information hotline, patient services, and vision screenings. Website has information on macular degeneration, an Amsler grid, and news about vision issues.

Women's Eye Health
Schepens Eye Research Institute
20 Staniford Street
Boston, MA 02114
617-573-3832
www.w-e-h.org

Coalition including the Schepens Eye Research Institute focusing on prevention of blindness in women. Information on lifestyle issues, children's eye exams, eye disease statistics among women, and eye exam checklists educate women on the gender risk factors of eye disease and how to provide adequate eye care for their families.

About the Authors

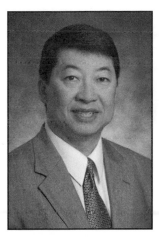

David F. Chang, MD, is a clinical professor of ophthalmology at the University of California, San Francisco, and has a private practice specializing in cataract surgery in Los Altos, California. Dr. Chang graduated from Harvard College and earned his Medical Degree from Harvard Medical School.

As an internationally acclaimed cataract expert, Dr. Chang has received the highest international awards for cataract surgery from the American Academy of Ophthalmology ([AAO] Kelman Lecture), the American Society of Cataract and Refractive Surgery ([ASCRS] Binkhorst Medal), the Asia-Pacific Association of Cataract & Refractive Surgeons (Lim Medal), the Canadian Society of Cataract and Refractive Surgery (Award of Excellence), the United Kingdom & Ireland Society of Cataract & Refractive Surgeons (Rayner Medal), the Indian Intraocular Implant & Refractive Society (Gold Medal), the Italian Society of Ophthalmology (Strampelli Medal), and the Royal Australia and New Zealand College of Ophthalmologists (Gregg Medal). He is the 2014 recipient of the Jose Rizal International Medal, the highest international award from the Asia-Pacific Academy of Ophthalmology.

Serving as president in 2012, Dr. Chang is on the executive board of ASCRS, the largest international specialty organization for cataract and refractive surgeons. He also chaired the AAO's national committee, which writes the clinical guidelines for cataract surgery that are used in the United States and in many foreign countries. Dr. Chang is co-chair of the ASCRS Foundation, and serves on the medical advisory board of 2 global humanitarian organizations: the Himalayan Cataract Project and Project Vision.

Dr. Chang is the author/editor of 4 best-selling books on cataract surgical techniques for ophthalmologists. *Mastering Refractive IOLs: The Art and Science* covers advanced lens implants, such as multifocal, pseudoaccommodating, and toric lenses, and is considered the most comprehensive textbook on the subject. He has served as Chief Medical Editor of *EyeWorld*, a leading trade journal that has a global circulation of more than 30,000 ophthalmologists. Dr. Chang is in the current national edition of *Best Doctors in America* and is listed by *Becker's* as one of the top 39 ophthalmologists in the United States.

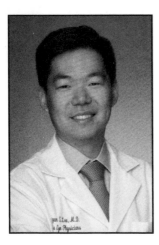

Bryan S. Lee, MD, JD, specializes in cataract, cornea, and refractive surgery at Altos Eye Physicians in Los Altos, California. Dr. Lee graduated magna cum laude from Harvard College and cum laude from Harvard Law School. He attended medical school at Washington University in St. Louis, Missouri, on a full merit scholarship and graduated with Alpha Omega Alpha honors.

Named one of the "Top 40 Under 40" in ophthalmology in 2015, Dr. Lee completed his ophthalmology residency at the Wilmer Eye Institute of Johns Hopkins. He was selected to receive further training in cornea, cataract, refractive, and glaucoma surgery at Minnesota Eye Consultants, one of the most prestigious fellowships in the country. While there, he was named Fellow of the Year by the Vanguard Ophthalmology Society.

Dr. Lee joined Altos Eye Physicians after spending 3 years as a cataract and cornea specialist on the faculty at the University of Washington. He received the Latham Vision Research Innovation Award for his academic pursuits, supervised the resident cornea clinic, and was selected to be the Washington Academy of Eye Physicians and Surgeons Speaker Series chair.

He is a leader in ophthalmology and serves on the Young Eye Surgeons committee of the American Society of Cataract and Refractive Surgery as well as on the Council of the American Academy of Ophthalmology (AAO). Dr. Lee served on the Washington and Maryland state eye society executive boards and is the secretary of the Vanguard Ophthalmology Society.

He has published dozens of peer-reviewed articles and textbook chapters and has taught multiple courses to other ophthalmologists. Dr. Lee also serves on the *EyeWorld* Cornea Section editorial board. His honors have included the AAO Achievement Award, Oliver Schein Research Grant Award, Walter J. Stark Research Grant Award, Maxwell Grand Prize for Excellence in Ophthalmology, and the Danforth and Distinguished Alumni Scholarships. In its first such survey, the international journal *The Ophthalmologist* selected Dr. Lee as one of the top 40 individuals in ophthalmology under the age of 40.

Index